Drink Water & Mind Your Business

Drink Water & Mind Your Business

A Black Woman's Guide to Unlearning the BS and Healing Your Self-Esteem

Dr. Donna Oriowo

sourcebooks

Copyright © 2025 by Dr. Donna Oriowo
Cover and internal design © 2025 by Sourcebooks
Cover design by Jillian Rahn/Sourcebooks
Cover images © AUDSHULE/Stocksy, Anastasiia Hevko/Getty Images, designer29/Getty Images
Internal design by Tara Jaggers/Sourcebooks
Internal images © Topuria Design/Getty Images, Bubaone/Getty Images

This publication is designed to provide accurate and authoritative information in regard to the subject matter covered. It is sold with the understanding that the publisher is not engaged in rendering legal, accounting, or other professional service. If legal advice or other expert assistance is required, the services of a competent professional person should be sought.—*From a Declaration of Principles Jointly Adopted by a Committee of the American Bar Association and a Committee of Publishers and Associations*

References to internet websites (URLs) were accurate at the time of writing. Neither the author nor Sourcebooks is responsible for URLs that may have expired or changed since the manuscript was prepared.

Published by Sourcebooks
P.O. Box 4410, Naperville, Illinois 60567-4410
(630) 961-3900
sourcebooks.com

Cataloging-in-Publication Data is on file with the Library of Congress.

Printed and bound in the United States of America.
VP 10 9 8 7 6 5 4 3 2 1

*"Don't expect to be healthy
when your oppressor is feeding you"*

To Black women, my first loves

For Bose, Felicia & Krystal

Contents

Foreword

The relationship we have with ourselves sets the stage for all others to follow. It's no wonder there's been so much research and attention dedicated to helping us cultivate a solid one. A large part of what shapes our relationship with ourselves is how we feel about ourselves and our capabilities, in short, our self-esteem. There are many factors that shape our self-esteem, including our experiences with childhood caregivers, friendships, romantic relationships, race, gender, country of origin, and socioeconomic status to name a few. And if we find ourselves at the intersection of Blackness and womanhood, there are likely some additional factors that become salient, including skin color, hair texture, and body features. While much attention has been paid to how self-esteem develops and what it looks like in other communities, far less attention has been given to how it develops and what it looks like in Black women, which is why the importance of this book cannot be understated.

Writing the foreword for this book has unlocked a very serendipitous and on-brand memory for me that I absolutely must share. I spent a part of my summer in 1998 as a budding young researcher on the campus of Emory University in Atlanta, GA. I had been accepted into the UNCF/Mellon Mays Undergraduate Fellowship designed for undergraduate students who were interested in pursuing a career in academia, so of course one of our first tasks was choosing a research question to explore and then setting out to design a study to answer that question. My question was "What is the relationship between skin color and self-esteem in Black women college students?" Now please forgive me because I do not remember much about this research project. I don't remember how many participants I had, what the findings were, or any of the juicy stuff. I do remember that I used the Rosenberg Self-Esteem Scale (RSE) to measure self-esteem in my participants, and I vaguely remember a navy blue folder that was used to contain all the papers I had for the project, but the rest is a blur. While it would be great to be able to remember more of the details about this very, very, very early work in my career, what feels most notable about this experience is that it marks a clear connecting point between my passion for Black women's mental health, the work I do today with Therapy for Black Girls, and this important body of work offered by Dr. Oriowo. It's like our paths connected before we even knew the other existed. At the very grown age of twenty, I had very little to contribute to the conversation about Black women's self-esteem and how it was developed, but thankfully twenty-plus years later, she has given us a magnificent starting point to dig deeper into this area both for ourselves and with those in our community.

As with much of the psychology and mental health field, the foundations for how we talk about self-esteem are largely based on a population that was not Black women. The RSE that I discussed earlier is probably the first instrument that was developed to measure self-esteem and was developed in 1979. Just think about what the world looked like then, and now think about what it looked like for Black women in particular. While some of the questions on the scale are fairly innocuous—I feel that I have a number of good qualities—it's not hard to imagine how responding to a statement like "I am able to do things as well as most other people" could be pretty layered depending on who you are and how you identify. Who are these other people? Do they make you feel welcomed in the environment? Do these other people share resources, or are they actively trying to sabotage your efforts? You get the point. If self-esteem is being measured by statements like these, we must take into consideration the larger context that exists, and sadly for far too long, this context has been absent. However, in *Drink Water and Mind Your Business*, that context is front and center. Not as an aside, but as central to our understanding of the concept. And not only is the context central; there are connections between self-esteem and other areas that I have not seen explored in this way, in any other literature. I was most moved by the connection Dr. Oriowo draws between self-esteem and sexuality. She makes it very clear that we often hear about how low self-esteem is linked to promiscuity, but what about how self-esteem is linked to pleasure? I've certainly not seen that explored elsewhere and enjoyed the connections made in this chapter about how the stories we're told about being "fast" as little girls impacts our self-esteem and ultimately our understanding of and ability to receive pleasure. I promise I won't spoil all the fun for you, but let me also just share one of my other favorite parts of the book, the connection between our self-talk and self-esteem. At a very basic level, it seems evident that of course how we talk to ourselves about ourselves is a reflection of our self-esteem, but the way in which she lays it out and connects it to love languages is both remarkable in its approach and easily accessible.

With *Drink Water and Mind Your Business*, Dr. Oriowo has given Black women both new ideas on how to think about the relationships we have cultivated with ourselves but also concrete strategies to improve the relationship. This work is a gift to Black women, people in relationships with us, and therapists holding space to help us heal. It brilliantly weaves theory with practice and provides the reader with an easy-to-follow journey of exploring what this thing called self-esteem is all about and how to improve it. I am grateful that Dr. Oriowo was bold enough to answer the call to share this work. We are all better for it. Wishing you care and gentleness as you begin your read. You are in good hands.

— **DR. JOY HARDEN BRADFORD**
Licensed psychologist and founder of Therapy for Black Girls
Author of *Sisterhood Heals: The Transformative Power of Healing In Community*

Introduction

I. LOVE. BLACK. WOMEN. I love the way we walk and talk. The way we show vulnerability and strength. The way we move into rooms. The way we birth ideas, products, smiles, and love. I love Black women. Not just because I am one (and it would be expected of me), but because of who we are in America and throughout the world.

What I don't like—what I don't love—is the ways in which the world around us has operated to hurt and keep us "in our place." What I don't appreciate is the way, from one generation to the next, traumas are passed on like heirlooms. What I don't like is that, because of the fucked-up world around us, we have internalized the belief that something is wrong with us. It's almost absurd to type—"something is wrong with us"—when we know a world built for rich white men could never and would never deign to be a world that sees us and accepts us for who we are. This may be why I so fiercely love Black women. The work I do centers us. I am a Black woman who serves Black women in all that I do.

And I am tired. I am tired of doing the most for the least, tired of not being seen, tired of the work it takes every day to be me in a world that shouts at me every day to conform. To give up what and who I am in order to fit into the boxes that they have created.

As a therapist, I am tired of seeing how the world beats down my clients the same way it has beaten me down. There is almost something primal about it. There is this need I have to protect Black women from the way these systems operate. To expose it, so we are aware. I talk about it all the time, but I never think folk really hear me, so I wanna say it here and to you. Let this introduction be the point of reference for everything you learn moving forward in this book and in how we all move forward in doing this healing work.

What you don't know: I am an avid reader and book lover. I am trying to grow a baby library in my house and in the Amazon cloud. I love Black women like that. Like a book. The front cover is beautiful and eye-catching, giving you the barest hints of what's inside. Much in the same way that my work calls to Black women. To say you are seen—in that regard, I serve as a therapist, teacher, friend, and a guide for free and at cost. Helping Black women along their story. On the back end, I have our backs. The anti-racism work I do with training organizations and corporations about diversity, equity, and inclusion is more about protecting all the loveliness that we are, than about helping them to meet invisible quotas and make false promises about how they will improve. I want change for our benefit. For our freedom and for our wellness. However, as will always be true, I know that my work will always start with us. Why? So that we are prepared to be in the spaces that are ready to receive us, so that we can help to cultivate those places that want us, and that when we get there, they know that "nobody puts Baby in a corner!"

Nice to Meet You!

Before we have even been properly introduced, you already know me to be tired. Yikes! So, let me backtrack on that. I want to introduce myself using the Johari window concept.

The Johari window is a visual framework you can use to identify and understand both your conscious and unconscious biases. It speaks to the truth of who we are and can help with developing self-awareness. The window model separates the self into four windowpanes: public, private, blind, and undiscovered. The **PUBLIC** self is what everyone can see, what you *allow* them to see. The **PRIVATE** self is not known to the public; it is only known to you and the few people you select to share it with. The **BLIND** self is what others can see and note about you but of which you are not aware, also known as *blind spots*. And the **UNDISCOVERED** self is simply that, undiscovered. It is information about you that has yet to be uncovered—maybe due to a lack of life experience or because you have not yet thought to explore other aspects of yourself. For whatever reason, it is closed off from you. For now.

JOHARI'S WINDOW

The PUBLIC Self What I and others BOTH see in me	**The PRIVATE Self** What I see but others do NOT see in me
The BLIND Self What others see but I do NOT see in me	**The UNDISCOVERED Self** What neither I nor others see in me

Normally, I would ask you to explore your public and private selves through values alone. However, we are here specifically to talk about your self-esteem.

✐ JOURNAL WORK

Think about your self-esteem and how it shows up in public spaces. How do you see and experience your self-esteem privately? And, if you're feeling brave, ask a friend, a family member, or just people you interact with semiregularly what they have noticed about how your self-esteem is expressed (or not expressed).

This gives us a starting point. In *Pleasure Activism* by Adrienne Maree Brown, I appreciated that the author began her story by introducing herself and her point of view. Introductions not only let you know someone's name, but they can help to build trust. And we are definitely gonna need some trust, especially for some of what I am gonna say here.

I am Dr. Donna Oladayo Oriowo. I am the daughter of two Nigerian immigrant parents who first immigrated to Belgium, tried on London for a day, went back to Belgium, and then came on over to America. I was born in Washington, DC, during a blizzard in early November. I was raised on jollof rice and mumbo sauce. I'm a product of DC and Maryland public schools. I lived with a grandma who was not my grandma, for a time. I have made and lost friends over time. I am telling you this bit because it gives you some context. You know how people talk about being unbiased? Well, it's a whole lie, and I can't start our new relationship, our journey together, based on a lie.

Here is my basic Johari window:

PUBLIC: I value authenticity, freedom, and self-esteem. But to be honest, I can't say I had high self-esteem growing up. I was more in the fake-it-'til-you-make-it club. My most memorable coming-into-self moment happened while writing my dissertation on texturism and realizing how much pain I was holding about my appearance. The process brought heightened anxiety, anger, and sorrow before healing made itself known. And I ain't done, because healing ain't a destination, nor is it finite.

PRIVATE: I find that I struggle with the space of how others see me and how I see myself. I have to remember what is and is not mine and come back to myself; when I do this, I feel at peace. There are always new levels to experiencing myself, and when I uncover them, I move back into anxiety before I get back to healing.

BLIND: Earlier I said that we cannot see this part of ourselves; it is based on the experience of others. So, it would seem ridiculous that I would have anything to add here. Except that I have asked. (Note: Ask others what they see in you *only* when you are ready to accept the fullness of their answer without blame and shame. It's okay to consider this and admit to yourself you're not yet ready.)

With regard to my self-esteem, I have been told that I present like I have it together but that I don't always give myself the credit for my "badassness." Another friend said: "I think you express your self-esteem by taking up space. I think sometimes people might not realize your struggles because you speak the language of someone with a really positive self-concept." Or, basically, my self-concept looks good out in the public space, but if they don't know, they don't know. I have been told that I am a person who appears to be self-absorbed. That I have high self-esteem but spend my time questioning it. That I present as a know-it-all—I have determined that this has more to do with my speaking in statements as opposed to having unstated question marks at the end of all my sentences—and that I can be abrasive.

Telling you all of this could feel really embarrassing, but in this moment, it doesn't. It just feels like the truth of who I am. I am a person who can and does struggle with separating my self-esteem from my worth defined by others, but I still know what I know and that we can make it through together. No one has it all together, so there is no need for me to present myself like I do. There will always be new levels the more we learn about ourselves and our place in the world. Healing is a constant practice, not a one and done. Like eating to sate your hunger, you must return to healing yourself as often as needed.

UNDISCOVERED: Still undiscovered.

Other info about me that may come up: I have a bachelor's degree in psychology, two master's degrees (one in social work and the other in education), and a doctorate degree in human sexuality. While these things often define a person's financial trajectory, they do not define who I am as a human being. That is me as the human doing—constantly on team Doin' Too Much.

My stance in this project:

→ I write this book in the knowledge and belief that white patri- archal, capitalist, heteronormative, supremacist delusion is the thing that has been oppressing us all and that no one actually benefits under its thumb. Not even the whites.

→ My experiences with sexism, racism, colorism, texturism, etc., have shaped a lot of how I see the world around me and have shaped the very nature of who I am.

→ Power is present in all relationships, including the one we have with ourselves, impacting how we feel, think, and behave.

→ *Healing* is a politically charged word that calls in the toxic nature of the systems we are involved in. So healing is also ongoing work, since the systems are ongoing.

→ I talk directly and specifically to Black women, but that doesn't mean other folk can't get something from this, too.

→ I cuss. A lot.

→ I believe that separation of concepts and ideas is an illusion that keeps us from gaining traction toward our actualized selves.

→ Pleasure and sexuality are often left out of conversations about self-esteem, and I think it's foolhardy and dangerous.

→ Change and growth are uncomfortable AF!

→ I am *a* therapist, not *your* therapist. Act accordingly.

→ I make no promises of healing your self-esteem. I take no responsibility for your healing. That is for you to do and for me to hope for.

Lastly, you need to be prepared. What I offer—and how I offer it—is truly based on who I am and the experiences I have had. It brings me pleasure to share with you what I know and what I have learned. I told you I wouldn't lie to you. I am telling it based on my eyes because the idea of objectivity is a whole-assed lie, and I don't want to pass it on in this book. That would be the opposite of bringing me pleasure, and it would be of little help to you. I am moving into this book as a Black, first-gen, eldest-daughter, sophisti-ratchet, DC-born, PG (pretty girl), county-raised, product-of-an-illustrious-HBCU (Morgan State), pansexual, married-to-a-Black-man, social-working, therapy-doing woman. These things color my experiences as well as the ways I talk, feel, and write about healing the self-esteem of Black women.

Part 1

MIND OVER MATTER

You Can't Solve the Problem You Don't (or Won't) See

I don't know about you, but all my life, when I came up to a roadblock, people would say, "Mind over matter." People making fun of you at school? "Don't mind them; mind over matter." Having a hard time grasping a taught concept? "Mind over matter." Feeling unwelcome or judged at work, and it's impacting how well you work? "Mind over matter." As far as the folk who use it like a prayer are concerned, using your full mind will make it so that any adversity doesn't matter. It's all in your head.

Can I be honest? I think *mind over matter*, quite frankly, is bull-shit. It's a false narrative akin to pulling yourself up by your bootstraps while not noting any of the conditions that may actively or passively prevent you from doing so. *Mind over matter* is a phrase that makes the systemic issue an individual one. Admittedly, I am still fond of this idiom. I use it here, both as a joke and as a request. The joke is in the fact that we know yelling at an armless, shoeless person will not help them to "pull themselves up by their bootstraps" any faster. I guess it's more ironic than funny. The request herein is that you, as my mother would say, "mind what you are doing" or "face your front." Lovingly known as the true *mind your business.*

We have to take care of that which is in front of us. But this requires us to have knowledge of what our business is. More to the point, what I'm saying here is that we need to make sure that we are taking the time to look back before we can go further into our goal of healing our own self-esteem.

When people talk about putting "mind over matter," they often fail to note that, in order to do so, you have to know the full parameters of what is going on; that's the only way you can understand exactly what it is that you need to overcome mentally in order to produce physical manifestations of that change. That is what I'm asking us to do now. Our first step in learning to put our mind over the matter of race, of sexuality, and of our self-esteem is to cultivate an in-depth knowledge of how we even got to this point—because as any therapist will tell you, the first step in being able to solve a problem is to *acknowledge* it.

For me, the second step is having a working operational definition of the problem, which includes knowing both its etymology and its etiology. To simplify: we gotta know the history, because context matters. In Ghana there is a word, *Sankofa,* which means "going back to move forward." We cannot go forward in the way that we choose without knowledge and acknowledgment of what has been, otherwise we may be doomed to repeat the past.

In Part 1, we will wholly define the problem—particularly, the problem of traditional self-help practices and how they fail to address the self-esteem of Black women. This is where we get a more robust understanding of what the problem is, so that we can place our minds over the matter of this foolishness. In other words, this is where we get *on top your matter.*

CHAPTER 1

What the Hell Is Self-Esteem, Anyway?

Who TF is Self-Esteem for?

I'm getting ahead of myself already because we haven't even defined *self-esteem*, but it's a question I want you to keep in mind as you read this chapter. Asking who self-esteem is for may seem like an odd question in the first place (doesn't everyone have self-esteem, good or bad?), but I promise it will make sense later.

Who TF Is This Book for?

This book is for Black women. I think the title may have already suggested that, but you know how people like to throw the word *Black* into the title for extra props with no actual substance. When I say *women*, I am talking about any Black self-identified woman. I don't care what you were born with; I care about who you know yourself to be. This is for any Black woman who has struggled with the idea of self-esteem. For the Black women who think about imposter syndrome in the workplace. For the Black women who wonder why they attract fuckfolk. This is for Black women who already look like they have it all together but feel a whole different way inside. This is for Black women who feel generally okay about where they are until they get into spaces with other people. This is for the Black women who could be your mom, sister, cousin, friend, enemy, stranger, and so forth. If you have felt the strain of self-esteem in big or small ways, I know this book will have something to offer you.

If your self-esteem depends on the money you have (or don't have) in the bank, the lightness or darkness of your skin, on what you look like, if it depends on if you have been "picked" for a relationship, on your job status, etc., then this book is for you. I already have you in mind. I am not gonna leave you out. This book is also for women of color and white women. Now, let me be real, if you're in that last category, I am not gonna talk directly to you, but that doesn't mean you can't benefit from this work. So, gather your shit, and let's take this journey together.

She Think This Book Special or Something?

Everybody thinks the thing they're doing is so unique and so special. And I am no different, sis! I got to thinking about what makes this work different. I admit, I do not have all the answers. I'm not here to sell you the idea that only I have the true key to good self-esteem. I won't pretend to be the only person with knowledge in this area or even to be *the* capital-*E Expert*. I think that is the height of arrogance, and I like to believe I'm not that arrogant—being Nigerian aside. Which means, for me, this needed to come with additional components. So, you will see that there are other therapists' definitions of self-esteem throughout this book as well as maybe a tip or two. And what I'd like you to do is also take some time to visit my website and watch the interviews. (Psst. The QR code to the right will take you there.) I think there's a lot to be gleaned from them. And certainly, it opens up the conversation to stop this idea of there being only one "right" way to know what self-esteem is and only one way to access it. I'm more interested in making sure that there are multiple routes to having the self-esteem that you want to have, however that looks. After all the saying is "There are many ways to skin a cat"—though I still don't know why we are skinning cats.

Another thing that makes this book different is that Black folk are the focus. Black people, and the unique challenges we face, are typically excluded. Black women in particular have been left out of all conversations about self-esteem. If *we* don't start that conversation, then we're not having it, because no one else is going to start that conversation for us. I am making sure that, for once, we are central in the way that we should have been in the first place. I'm centering the Black woman's experience and how we are able to access all that self-esteem greatness.

A Book Is Not a People!

This isn't a book made for my proselytizing (*though if you want me to pass the collection plate, I will*). There are actual steps that I want you to take from this book. Which means we're not just reading to read. We're reading for life. We're reading for change. We're reading so we can actually understand, access, and heal our self-esteem.

ICYMI: Healing is not a destination; it is not linear. Healing is a whole-assed journey that has ups and downs—which can sometimes make you feel like you're moving backwards or even not moving at all. It can be hard out there in them healing streets. The other thing to remember/consider is this: If you weren't harmed in isolation, why would healing be a solo job? Healing happens in community. Meaning this work is not just for you by yourself. It's also for your friends, your sisters, your comrades in arms, your badass bitch group, and anyone you know whose self-esteem is compromised.

These folk will be very important in your healing journey, because you need someone who has your back and will hold you accountable. You will learn from each other. And because healing and stepping into your authentic self requires vulnerability, your community can help you build up that muscle of showing up as you and allowing space for you to stand in the truth of who you are. So, start a book club or whatever you need to make sure you know that you are not alone in doing this work.

Look, me and this book are only here for a small portion of your life. And I don't even know you like that! This is why you need people who have been there and will be there longer. People who will love you through the nonlinear healing process that continues throughout your lifespan. The book can be a part of that journey, but this book is not a person. I am a distant part of your tribe. I want you to build with people who love you up close.

Self-Esteem: It's a Vibe

I've said it before, and I'm gonna say it again: there is no problem that can be resolved if we don't acknowledge it as a problem and then work to define it.

Let's start with the basics. According to *Merriam-Webster Dictionary*, *self-esteem* is defined as

1. a confidence and satisfaction in oneself: **self-respect**
2. **self-conceit**

Did this answer what self-esteem is? Probably not. Because this definition lacks nuance and context—even if it does accurately cover the basis of self-esteem. Let me give you more with a little Psych 101, some developmental psychology, and a tad of my inner social worker to really dig into the *full* definition of self-esteem.

☕ *IT'S TEA TIME!*

Don't tell nobody, but back in the day when I was in middle school or so, I was doing homework in my shared room, on my bed. Now, we had an aunt (not of blood relation) staying with us at the time. Please remember: I am the firstborn daughter of immigrants. What I knew of myself was that I was meant to be a child who does as they are told, who gets good grades, and who sets a good example for my younger sisters.

Now, you see how my self-concept was set in those three things. I wanted to be a good daughter and that is what needed to happen to be considered one. And, so far so good—even if my grades weren't the best.

One day, my aunt said to me: "Get down here and clean this room." My mom had *just* told me to do my homework, so doing what I was told and getting good grades were now in direct conflict with each other. But my mom had seniority, so I said:

"I will clean it right after I am done with my homework."

Now, to someone not trying to exert power over someone else, in their home, while standing in their room, this might have seemed reasonable. But when you are feeling low, sometimes you wanna kick someone so they will feel lower (relational self-esteem). So, while what I said was fine, she probably heard:

"I'll do it when I feel like it."

To which she then responded: "Do it now."

What I heard was, "I don't give a damn if you fail; you gon' do what TF I just said."

So, I repeated: "When I am done." The "bitch" at the end of my sentence was silent, but damn it she HEARD IT in my attitude!

So, she slapped me. And I...SLAPPED HER BACK!

She was aghast, and I was shocked and shooketh!

What the hell had I just done? My actions and my words were out of alignment with the self-concept I was told was okay for me to have.

I was out of pocket and my ass was gonna be on fire!

But the conversation with my mom didn't go the way you would expect—you know, less talking and more belt. No, instead she told me that I was right, but that I shouldn't hit adults. My momma told me, "You're smarter than most adults."

Now, what do you think this did my to my self-concept? How about my self-esteem?

FIRSTLY, SELF-ESTEEM IS HOW A PERSON FEELS ABOUT THEM-SELF, THEIR WORTH, OR THEIR VALUE. (And this includes how much you like or appreciate yourself.) *Self-esteem* is defined by the presence of many elements—some of which include self-confidence, identity, sense of belonging, and self-competence. However, self-esteem is also about how we relate to others, the abilities we have, and how we feel about all of these factors in comparison to others. I know, it can feel wild that self-esteem still ends up being about someone else, even if that component is marginal. However, the part where others are involved is not just what they think about you, but rather what *you* think they think about you. Got it? If not, don't worry, there's more.

There are many schools of thought around self-esteem, and when people talk about it, they use many different words to describe it (e.g., *self-worth*, *self-regard*, *self-respect*). And, often, these terms are used interchangeably. But we won't do that here because words mean things. Let me break it down.

Look at the word *esteem*. What does this word mean to you? Personally, when I think about *esteem*, I think about respect, holding someone in admiration or high regard. We might also think about someone who is liked, admired, or valued. That person who we hold in esteem might be someone who is thought highly of or who we even have some reverence for. I think about Nina Simone, Maya Angelou, Angela Bassett, Luvvie Ajayi Jones, Sonya Renee Taylor, and Yvonne Orji, to name a few you might recognize. I also think about people I know on a more personal level like Dr. Lexx Brown-James, Dr. Joy Harden Bradford, Dr. Shamyra Howard, Ericka Hart, and Sonalee Rashatwar. When I hold someone in the highest *esteem*, it means that there is a quality about them that I recognize, value, and admire.

Let's do a quick exercise. Consider some folk you hold in high esteem and spend some time thinking about what trait(s) they have that you admire and why.

✍ JOURNAL WORK

Grab a piece of paper and draw three columns. Label them left-to-right as "Name of Person," "Admired Esteem Trait," and "Why Do You Admire It?" In the first column, list the names of people you hold in high esteem. In the second column, identify which traits you admire for each of those people. And in the third column, explain why you admire those traits. When we put the *self* back in with *esteem,* we can more clearly see how self-esteem is about how we admire, regard, appreciate, value, and respect ourselves.

Let's head back to our main definition of *self-esteem.* I said earlier, there are lots of words that are used interchangeably to describe self-esteem. It seems to not be about esteem alone. It's also about how all the other ideas about self-esteem intertwine with one another to create the you that you are when you're around other people. *And* it shapes how you are when you are alone. In a self-esteem checkup or quiz, you would see they ask about self-satisfaction, self-respect, and also how you feel about yourself in relation to others. Example: "I like myself, even when others reject me" or "I am as valuable a person as anyone else." Basically, self-esteem is a *vibe*.

"But what if she conceited, though?!" Remember, self-esteem is not just about how you vibe on your own, but also how others catch the vibe. When folk talk about someone who is conceited, we are basically saying that someone thinks that they're God's gift to humanity. They are too confident, too full of themselves. But even self-conceit is not just about them; it's also about how they are perceived and received. One person's confidence can be another person's conceit; it's all a matter of perspective. It can feel quite confusing for the definition to go from self-confidence and -satisfaction to self-conceit, all while being housed under the umbrella of self-esteem. It can feel like the line between self-esteem and -conceit is blurred. I don't know about you, but it would have me asking, "Well, how do I know when I have moved from esteem in myself to being conceited? Is being conceited always a bad thing? What counts as conceit? And who gets to judge that I have moved from being a person with esteem to a person who is conceited?!"

These are all good questions. And here is the thing: sometimes people who are pretty low on themselves may receive your confidence as conceit. And other times your behavior can be harmful to the point that people can only think that you believe you are better or more valued than them...which is conceited.

See, this is why we are having this conversation about what self-esteem is and isn't (or whatever, 'cause this a book). There is so much confusion about self-esteem and what's involved, but the whole conversation is kind of moot. In reality, if it's about you and it impacts the way you see, feel, express, and value yourself, chances are it is one of the major components of who you are and should have some level of consideration with how you personally choose to define self-esteem.

Confidence, self-satisfaction, self-respect, etc., are all separate concepts. They complement one another, but they are not the same thing, much like your thoughts and emotions are not the same and yet can be so closely related that it can be hard to tell what you're thinking and separate it from what you're feeling. These ideas that are used interchangeably are separate, but they all go toward your self-concept.

SELF-CONCEPT INCLUDES EVERYTHING THERE IS TO KNOW ABOUT YOU: YOUR BELIEFS, ABILITIES, QUALITIES, AND REGULAR DAILY BEHAVIORS. Carl Rogers, the psychologist who talks about self-esteem as a theory, would say that self-esteem is a component of your self-concept.[1] Oftentimes, when we are thinking about self-esteem (that is, how we feel about ourselves), we are including our general self-concept. This is why it can be so hard to pin down an understanding, if not a definition, of *self-esteem*. This merging of the two ideas is also why there is so much divergence in what folk are referring to when they are talking about self-esteem. There are just so many interrelated concepts from various theorists over the years that it's hard for people to leave anything out. Using my business as the example: Concept = good, obedient Nigerian eldest daughter. Esteem = how I feel about my role as a good, obedient Nigerian eldest daughter.

Our first ideas of self-esteem come from our parents, and whether or not we're living up to their idea of who they think we should be.[2] I know there's a lot to unpack when it comes to parental relationships, so don't worry, we will cover more of this later. The point is that your self-esteem and -concept are not created in a bubble; they are created in context with others and start, oftentimes, with our caregivers or parents.

☕ MORE TEA TIME!

Both my aunt and I were rocked that day when I hit her back. The conversation with my mom kept me rocking, because, suddenly, I no longer needed to do what I was told—I am, after all, smarter. And, being a preteen, I completely dropped the admonishment for hitting my aunt and only heard that I was right for doing my homework and giving my explanation. This was the day my self-concept shifted. And I wasn't quite sure how to feel about it at first. I knew how to do what I was told. I didn't know how to make my own rules as a pseudo-adult. *But don't worry, I found my way...*

If your parents, for example, don't meet your needs when you are a baby, this can foster mistrust. If they don't feed you when you need to be fed, hold you when you need to be held, or change you when you need to be changed, trust is out the window, and everything looks suspect. You might grow up thinking and feeling like other people are not reliable or trustworthy and have no real memory of where that even started. It can look like extreme self-reliance or independence, which can come off as being conceited or arrogant.

See? I told you self-esteem is based on what messages you receive from others that foster love and support, your actual abilities and competency to do things, and how you see yourself and your abilities in comparison to others. It's also why it can feel like it fluctuates and is not the stable concept that people say it should be when you *really* love yourself. But look at what was just said: what your parents/caregivers did (or didn't do) as you grew impacts that very concept of self! Now let's talk about the flip side, if your parents did meet your needs, this can foster a sense of trust and self-confidence in your abilities, which can translate into how you develop from a child to an adult with maybe more stable self-esteem...or conceit, depending on who you talk to. ;)

✐ JOURNAL WORK

SPHERE OF INFLUENCE
Grab your journal and write out everything that you feel has impacted your self-esteem.

Here's the thing: if the concepts aren't really separate, and if they also talk about you in relation to other people, then how can self-esteem or even self-concept be built by yourself? *It can't.* It doesn't make any sense. However, Western ways of considering the individual as someone who needs to "pull themselves up by their bootstraps" permeate the space of self-esteem and self-concept. It makes it solely a *you* thing, instead of considering how it's more of a *we* thing. Think about it: I just told you that your parents make a huge freaking difference. But also consider this: What happens when you are Black, and the world has proven itself untrustworthy? Or when you are a woman, and the world has confirmed it doesn't value you nearly as much as it does someone with a penis who identifies as male? This is also why all of these concepts, as lovely as they are, can feel so incomplete, because there are all of these people talking about self-esteem and lived experiences, but where is the consideration for the lived experience of the Black woman, a person at the intersection of being undervalued by way of race *and* sex? This is why I say…

SELF-ESTEEM IS FOR WHITE PEOPLE

…or, rather, that is what it can look like. Especially given that so many of the self-esteem books out here in these streets almost treat race and the intersection with gender as an ancillary happenstance.

What Is Really Affected by Self-Esteem?

Short answer: errything. But let's rewind a little. Have you noticed the way some folk talk about self-esteem? They talk about it like it barely matters. That what really matters is making yourself do what you have to do because "it is what it is." Whew, that whole saying really gets on my damn nerves.

Back to the question, there is not one area of your life that is not or will not be impacted by your self-esteem, self-efficacy, and self-concept. Ain't no way for it not to be. We already talked about self-concept being about everything that there is to know about Y-O-U. You take yourself and your history into every room you enter. Self-esteem shows up in every conversation you have, every outfit you pick out, every person you kiss or have sex with. It shows up in every choice you make and the ones you don't make due to fear. It shows up in how others treat you and how you treat others, what your boundaries are, and if you even have boundaries in the first, second, and third place. Your self-esteem and self-concept are ever present, periodt.

FYI, if you skipped my introduction, then you may not know that I am a sex and relationship therapist. Which means you are gonna be hella confused when I start talking about sex and self-esteem. So, I am warning you now, again, we will talk about how self-esteem shows up in relationships, in sex, and in mental health as a whole. Mmmmk?

CHAPTER 2

What Makes Up Self-Esteem?

Alright, so now we know what self-esteem is in the context of this book and how it is different from self-concept. If you missed it before: self-esteem = how we *feel* about ourselves, and self-concept = what we *know* about ourselves. BOOM!

A definition only gets us so far, though. We still need more information about what makes up self-esteem. Think about *The Powerpuff Girls* (Buttercup, Bubbles, and Blossom). Hopefully you know what I am talking about. In the show's theme song, a voiceover recites the recipe the professor used when he made them. The ingredients for the "perfect little girls" are sugar, spice, and everything nice. And because he wasn't paying attention (or he's as clumsy as I can be), he knocked some chemical X into the batch and got the kick-ass, crime-fighting Powerpuff Girls instead. Flyana Boss in the "You Wish" music video, on the other hand, has me feeling made of sugar, spice, Kanekalon, and cinnamon.

Okay, if you're on the younger side, you may have no idea WTF I am talking about. No problem! Instead, think about what you need to make some amazing-assed chicken, cornbread, or jollof rice. There are ingredients you need that must be added in specific quantities for it to taste right and not make the fam revoke your right to bring anything other than paper plates to the next family function. Well, self-esteem isn't much different. There are all kinds of things that end up in it to make it what it is. The ingredients that make up self-esteem, just like jollof rice, change depending on who you are talking to and when you are talking to them. There are jollof wars for a reason. The way Nigerians, Ghanaians, and Gambians each make jollof rice is different. Different histories and context go into the process. Same goes for what ingredients that make up self-esteem.

Some of the components for self-esteem include:

→ Reactions of others to you
→ Experiences
→ Illness/disability/injury
→ Age, role, and status in society
→ Media messaging
→ Thoughts and perceptions
→ Self-confidence
→ Feelings of security
→ Identity
→ Sense of belonging
→ Competence/incompetence
→ Self-efficacy
→ Self-respect
→ Compassion for others and your ideal self

→ Identity
→ Appreciation
→ Acceptance
→ Pride
→ Humility
→ Selfishness
→ Security
→ Sense of purpose
→ Trusting and being trusted
→ Contribution
→ Influence
→ Self-control

→ Sense of family pride
→ Sense of reward
→ Self-love
→ Self-worth
→ Messages of love, support, and approval
→ Role and status in society
→ Thoughts, perceptions, and experiences
→ The way you regard specific aspects of yourself

This is a list-list, okay! While I tried my best not to repeat things, many of the concepts greatly overlap or even feel like they are getting to the same thing. The point here is that a good chunk of them are about *your perceptions*—how you see things—while the other part of the list is how others treat you. There! Proof that self-esteem is not self-taught, self-cultivated, or self-built!

Even with all the diversity in the list of what the components are, it doesn't mean that anyone is wrong—except with what goes in jollof rice because everyone knows Nigerian jollof is the only one that counts—but with self-esteem, the various views and items on the list only add to our understanding of (*okay, and our confusion about)* the concept as a whole. But one thing that I read stood out among the rest: self-esteem components differ according to what we each find to be important.[1]

Don't miss that gem! I will say it again in case you did:

THE COMPONENTS TO SELF-ESTEEM WILL BE DIFFERENT TO WHAT WE EACH FIND TO BE IMPORTANT.

That means **YOU** choose the components that are important to you for **YOUR** self-esteem! But how to do it? And how do we know if what we choose as our components will lead to high or low self-esteem?

In this chapter, we are going to explore the highs and lows of self-esteem, go through the building blocks, and talk about self-esteem as it relates to Maslow's hierarchy of needs. The goal is to give us an understanding of self-esteem and what goes into it from different perspectives. While I think there are some steps in between, knowledge of the problem's full scope definitely adds to our ability to later do better. Let's get into that knowledge!

You're Either *the* Shit or *Some* Shit: The Highs and Lows of Self-Esteem

This seems like a great place to start, especially since you have to get to choosing what you're adding to your self-esteem pot.

As it stands, a lot of us think about self-esteem in terms of high or low, either being *the* shit or feeling like *some* shit. Almost like good or bad—either you have good self-esteem (and it tastes great like Naija jollof) or you have bad self-esteem (like jollof made with raisins as a feature). Sometimes we think of it as an either-or. Like either you got it, or you don't. But sunshine, I don't know if that is accurate, or at least not entirely accurate. It is very rare that something is easily defined in those binary terms. The more you study something, the more you see that it's on a spectrum rather than a binary. Think about it, some of us have been taught sex on a binary. You are either female or male. But let me tell you, studying sexuality in school taught me that even that is on a spectrum because intersex people exist—and their "maleness" or "femaleness" can vary! They aren't any *one* thing; they are both and neither at the same damn time! Who we are is so much more than our genitals, hormones, and gonads. Self-esteem is no different; it doesn't run on a binary either.

Why You Gotta Be So Insecure?

I know I just said that self-esteem is not on a binary, but let's start with the binary and expand out. There are researchers who talk about self-esteem a bit differently. Not like you have it or you don't. More like, we all have it, but it might feel secure or hella insecure (a.k.a. fragile). **SECURE SELF-ESTEEM** is a steadier view of yourself because it's based on what you *know* and what you *feel* about yourself. It doesn't rely on what other people think about you, so it doesn't fluctuate a lot. **FRAGILE SELF-ESTEEM**, on the other hand, is much more dependent on others. It's like living your life for the compliments, constantly looking for validation from other people. Insecure (fragile) self-esteem also has a basis in an insecure attachment style. Basically, you spend much of your time needing and seeking validation that you are *the* shit. This makes it so that everyone around you ends up with the job of placating your need for validation, but *you* still hardly believe them. So, you exhaust yourself doing *the most* to make sure the people you are in a relationship with (romantic, platonic, work, etc.) will stay thinking and proclaiming you as being *the* shit. The problem is you end up feeling like just plain ol' shit due to copious amounts of anxiety, which often shows up as perfectionism and people-pleasing. You try to be the perfect partner, the perfect employee, the perfect everything. Because your self-esteem is so fragile, any type of feedback that isn't about your greatness would come to you through that fragile lens and be interpreted as though *you* are a bad or damaged person, as opposed to simply, "Here is something we need to see improved on."

⌘ JOURNAL WORK

If you are expected to be perfect in all areas of your life, what do you expect from others? How does it impact your relationships with others who have to experience this perfection? I once asked this question in the therapy room and on social media. But this is something for you to consider if perfectionism is your constant companion.

It's funny (not *ha-ha*, but rather *peculiar*) because, as a therapist and an educator helping Black women feel *Free, Fabulous, and Fucked*, I see plenty of people who swear they have high (or secure) self-esteem, but the second I give them feedback on something they could have done differently, it all goes to hell. You would have thought I said they were ugly or that I slapped their mama! But this is also where fixed and growth mindset come in. Folk with secure self-esteem are more likely to have a **GROWTH MINDSET**—a tendency to believe that you start in one place but can improve as you learn. I think of it as, they learn better, so they have an opportunity to try and do better. Folk with low (or fragile) self-esteem are more likely to have a **FIXED MINDSET**—a tendency to believe that you are as good as you're gonna get, so what you display naturally is the limit of your skills. A fixed mindset can make a person believe that they have to do "it" right and be perfect the first time. Not to mention that folk who have fragile self-esteem are less likely to try new things because they don't want to fail at them. *Ain't that some shit?*

Hell, it also makes me think of romantic relationships. When we break up with someone, some of us act like we failed the relationship instead of thinking that maybe we were simply not right for each other at that time. With a growth mindset, you would look at the relationship, see where you might have fucked up, see where they might have fucked up, and take it as a lesson to use in your next relationship. That fixed mindset, however, will have your ass either saying it was all their fault (so you can protect your ego), or it will have you on some "I failed it by myself; I am broken" type shit. It doesn't allow you space to see things as they are, so you paint yourself (or them) with a brush of fuckedupness. So, then you might say, "There is nothing but pee and trash in the dating pool," and you never look to be in a relationship again, closing off emotionally, while simultaneously sitting in the therapy chair telling me how you want to date, yet you never leave your house and don't use dating apps, and I keep saying, "Ma'am, you are emotionally unavailable!" But I digress. The point is that fragile self-esteem, with its ties to a fixed mindset, means it's hard to see a full and accurate picture of what happened so you can move on without the steamer trunk of nonsense.

Anyway, back to our regularly scheduled programming.

What I was saying is that self-esteem is not on a binary of "you have it" or "you don't have it." We all have self-esteem; we just may not have *secure* self-esteem every moment of every day. It's more like a categorized spectrum. Lemme show you:

Secure Self-Esteem	Steady self view and evaluations
Fragile (Insecure) High Self-Esteem	High on performance or evaluations, with unrealistic self views and consistently seeking external validation
Damaged Self-Esteem	You see/say your esteem is low, but deep inside you actually have high internal self-esteem. This one is said to be about a disturbance in early development
Low Stable Self-esteem	Not seeking external validation because you don't think you'll get it, and low internal self-esteem cuz you ain't got it

This spectrum shows you some of the concepts I previously explained, but it also adds the ideas of **DAMAGED SELF-ESTEEM** and **LOW STABLE SELF-ESTEEM** to the mix. Damaged self-esteem occurs when, on the inside, you low-key like yourself—high self-esteem—but something happened (or keeps happening) that makes you doubt if you should, or feel like you're judging it wrong. So, if someone asked you, you'd say it's low. Low stable self-esteem on the other hand, is like you not seeing much of anything to like about yourself and feeling like, yup, the world just confirmed it. They just don't feel stable self-esteem, almost ever.

The thing is, so much about self-esteem is also based on attachment styles. **ATTACHMENT STYLES**, at their core, are about how we relate to other people and how our relationship develops based on previous experiences. Now, I know you may have heard about it, even if you don't know the nitty-gritty. Well, Imma be straight with you, I will NOT be giving you the nitty-gritty. But I will give you an overview as I once explained it to a client. Then you can go read *Polysecure* by Jessica Fern or something—it goes very in-depth about attachment styles.

Secure	"I am great; you are great"
Anxious/ Preoccupied	"I hope you like me" "I think I am the problem here; I'll fix it"
Dismissive/ Avoidant:	"I am not gonna be vulnerable" "The problem isn't me" "Imma be in this relationship, but Imma do me"
Fearful/Avoidant	"These hoes ain't loyal...so I won't get into a relationship because I can't be vulnerable to people who won't be loyal to me"

The (very) basic premise here is that when you are operating from a secure standpoint, you are also more likely to exhibit high secure self-esteem. When we start getting to the anxious, dismissive, and fearful attachment styles, one of the other types of self-esteem are more present.

But here's the thing, some people talk about attachment styles as finite, done, in the past, and based on your parents, with no hope for something different. Those people would be wrong. The truth is that your attachment style *can* change with intentional work! So, no worries. You are not doomed because of the starting place you inherited. You have the power to change it, but you have to possess the will to change it.

Snickers once said, "You're not you when you're hungry." The same is true when you have fragile self-esteem. You are literally trying to be whatever other people want so that you can be praised as the best in relation to those other people—a.k.a. so you can stop being hungry...or thirsty. You want to be the best partner, child, mother, worker, etc., so you are constantly seeking perfection because your high is from the praise. You may not low-key even know who you are without others telling you with compliments.

The problem is when others give you feedback or criticize something you have done, you take it as a strike against your character and who you are at your core, and then you can be put right back into a state of self-esteem famine. That's why it is called *fragile*. It's controlled more by the words and actions of others than it is by you. I personally think this is where shame lives. While guilt tells us that we may have done something wrong, it still gives us room to evaluate, and we can use our growth mindset to make a different choice in the future. Shame, however, tells us that something is wrong with us and that we have to do a better job of hiding it or else people will know and shun us or throw shit at us in the streets. But that's the thing; we are worried about *rejection*. Whether or not we will still be part of a family, a work environment, or any one of our communities. Basically, when self-esteem is fragile, you can be *defensive AF* because you're scared you're going to be booted off the island. It can make us desperate for people to like and accept us—even if we don't even like those people.

And for all my love of Black women, I think that a lot of us actually have fragile and damaged self-esteem. We know what self-esteem is "supposed" to look like, so we employ the fake-it-'til-you-make-it method. Here is the thing though, some of us would never self-categorize as having fragile or damaged self-esteem. Some of us wouldn't even say it out loud that we're unsure of our attachment style, because we are too scared and ashamed to examine it and accidentally let other people know that how we feel about ourselves is not secure but rather fragile AF. But we don't want people to know, so we cover it up with the shit that we buy, the trips that we take, and the people we date.

Regardless of what category you are in self-esteem wise, what we know to be true is that you can always make moves. If you are in a space where you have fragile self-esteem or damaged self-esteem, you can move to secure self-esteem. And for the purposes of this book: **THAT'S THE POINT**. The point is that a lot of us are operating in this insecure high self-esteem space (i.e., fragile self-esteem); some of us are also in that damaged self-esteem space where internally we have high self-esteem, but externally we display some low shit. I'm saying that we can all move to secure self-esteem, but first we got to call a motherfucking spade a spade.

Instead, we are stuck on the fake-it-'til-you-make-it train and my question is: Do we want to stay there, or do we want to move? If you want to move, then I will see you in the next section. If you are satisfied with where you are…I guess you can stop here.

✍ (NOT SO) QUICK JOURNAL WORK

Consider which self-esteem you have primarily. What and when does it change? What are some of the components that are currently making up your self-esteem and what components do you want to make up your self-esteem?

Get Your Shit Together! Worth, Love, and Growing

Now you know what makes up self-esteem for you and even what kind you have and when, it's time we get into what Glen R. Schiraldi knows.[2] Schiraldi discusses a clear order to follow as you grow your self-esteem. In the first stage of this process, you must adopt a sense of unconditional worth for yourself; in the second stage, you develop love for yourself; and in the third and final stage, the growing happens. Seems simple enough, right? But what I see is this: our access to stable secure self-esteem suffers because we have shaky worth at best, love that we barely understand, and growing that we value before anything else is firmly in place. Black folk are taught to shine first and foremost because we are looked at as being inherently worthless. How we look and come off to others becomes primary. So, we place the emphasis there before we really know ourselves and can learn to like it.

UNCONDITIONAL WORTH

Unconditional worth is almost exactly what it sounds like. You can see and experience your worth without feeling that you have to change anything about yourself or even do anything to get it. You already have it, simply because YOU. ARE.

Now, if you are churchy, the idea that God knew you, and *all* the bullshit you were gonna get into, and loves you still, should sound familiar. You can't earn God's love, and you can't do anything to un-earn it. Issa gift. No refunds or exchanges, no matter what you do. That's what's meant by unconditional. It has...no conditions!

This means regardless of what you do (or don't) believe, you have worth because you exist. Dassit! Your worth is unconditional. Now, your actions may be subject to being evaluated as good and worthy or bad and unworthy—with all the rewards or consequences that come with it. However, you as a person, regardless of your actions, already have internal cain't-no-one-take-that-shit-because-YOU-ARE **WORTH**!

Our worth, one human to another human, is the same. Period.

ASK ME HOW I KNOW!

I know because they are human just like you. I know because they bleed red, eat food, and take shits. No one sitting on the toilet looks that great while having a bowel movement. We are all people, and that gives us equal worth.

You already had everything you needed when you were born. Yes, there was some growing to do and some experiences to have, and those things do mold you, but your worth was already there from the start. Coloring, height, experiences, etc., don't mean much outside of how the world decides to treat people with similar or dissimilar experiences and looks. Don't get me wrong; we can't dismiss the bullshit ways folks are treated, but we also need to know that despite the treatment, you are of worth!

SO, WHAT DO YOU BRING TO THE TABLE?

The problem is we are often surrounded by people (and have been indoctrinated) in a world that sees worth as being very much related to money in the bank or assets acquired. It can be hard to see ourselves outside of monetary gain and usefulness. People want someone who is "worth" something to them—so basically someone who is of service. Which is why fuckfolk stay asking, "What do you bring to the table?" When our worth is based on our relative use to others, we have to prove ourselves to be useful, prove that we are deserving of payment, of housing, of food, of safety, prove that our bodies and minds can be used to their advantage. Or if all else fails, we prove our worth by how much cotton we have in the bank.

As a culture, we like to play around with the word *unconditional*, but we don't actually like to practice it. And I get it; it feels a bit unwieldy. For something to truly be unconditional, there can't be any conditions or terms that must be met before it is enacted. That's a lot to ask of people, especially as our world tries to tell us that people with more money are worth more. (That ain't true. They *have* more. They aren't *worth* more.) Our world also tries to tell us that white people are better than Black people and people of color, and that men are better than women, that light-skinned people are better and thus worth more than darker-skinned people, that cis and straight people are better than trans and queer folk. But again, this is not true. They may have more privilege in a world that favors them, but their worth is equal to your worth. Not greater, not lesser. Just the same. Our efforts are a whole other conversation.

But what they think of you, while important-ish, will never fill your cup. You may get a sense of esteem from them, but your self-esteem cup will remain empty because only you can fill it.

In Sonya Renee Taylor's book *The Body Is Not An Apology*, she talks about worth. She claims that worth is innate and that we are prone to radical self-love but that external factors—the way our world functions—get in the way of our "purpose and destiny." She uses an acorn as an example. The acorn has a purpose and a destiny: to one day become an oak tree. It doesn't need to understand much more than its purpose in order to make it happen. So, this is the idea of you being complete—having everything you need to reach your highest self, or self-actualization, but you are not completed, as in you aren't an oak tree, yet.

The thing is, an acorn may be unobstructed in its ability to become an oak tree. But Black women are not unobstructed from embodying our highest selves. No, we are obstructed by the white and male supremacist delusions that exact control by limiting our options. One way they do this is by taking our innate unconditional worth and replacing it with conditional worth, creating terms that are inhospitable for meeting our purpose and destiny. We can know what and who we are, but in an environment made for only the willow tree to thrive, we barely are hanging on.

So, what have we done? Adapted. We become less oak and more willow in order to survive. We are taught that projecting a willow facade will ensure jobs, housing, and general well-being, despite evidence to the contrary. We try our best, but it's hard for us to reach our full potential when we are emulating people who are, high-key, copying us. The adaptation with respectability politics at the center means survival but at the cost of what we could have been if we were being us. But I get it though, sometimes being your authentic self has consequences. And I don't know about you, but I like eating a few meals a day and having a roof over my head and clothes I chose on my back. So sometimes, we compromise as a survival method and harm ourselves simultaneously.

The point is this: you have innate worth, even if others don't see it or value it. What would happen if we saw our individual worth outside of material factors and believed that we have unconditional worth at our core? Well, we might get to Schiraldi's second stage.

LOVE.

Once you embrace your unconditional worth, it's easier to find things about yourself to like. You can like these things outside of what other people think and not compare them. But Schiraldi talks about LOVE, not just like.[3] *Amore!* And love is, according to the dictionary, "an intense feeling of deep affection," "a great interest or pleasure in something," "to hold dear; cherish," or "to like or desire actively."

Bay-bee, there is a lot to be said about it and around it.

Is this all love is? Deep affection? Well, we know that when you ask a question, many will answer. Talking about love is no different. I read something that said love isn't an emotion at all, but more like a drive, kind of like hunger.[4] Others say love is made up of a bunch of different emotions, actions, and choices. As for the purpose of this text, I am taking a both/and kind of approach. Love is an emotion, made up of other emotions, that is shown through actions and choices. This means that I will use Robert Sternberg's triangular theory of love, which says there are three components that make up love: passion, intimacy, and commitment.

Passion is the type of enthusiasm that can move you to action. Intimacy makes me think of how some of my therapist friends will say, "Into me you see," or the culture of your relationship, as my good friend Goody Howard (@askgoody) would say. And commitment is, according to *Merriam-Webster Dictionary*, your pledge, agreement, or obligation to something—the something is *love*.

From these three ingredients, you can get seven types of love. Some of these types have one ingredient, others have two, and the final one has all three.

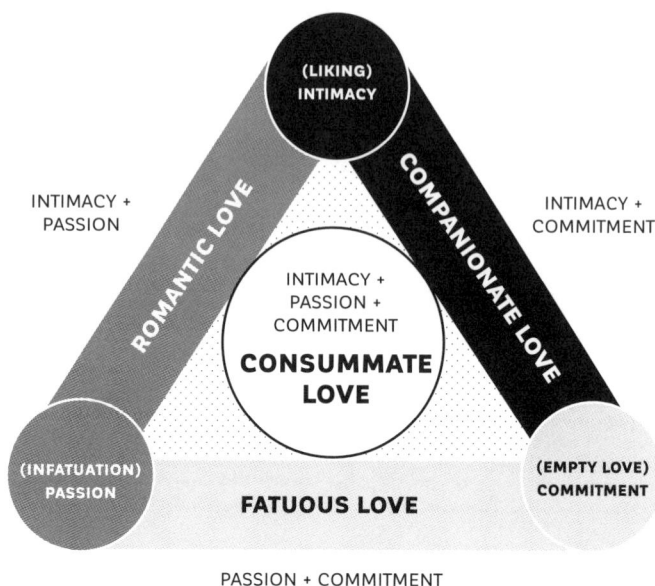

Why mention all this? Because there are many ways we can love ourselves. As we understand our worth and value over time, how we love ourselves can change. It can be empty love (**COMMITMENT**—you are in your body and dassit). You can like yourself without having a commitment to yourself (**INTIMACY**), and you can have infatuation or an intense drive for yourself that burns out with time (**PASSION**). Ain't nothing wrong with any of these types of love. They all have a reason and a season. This is love in the context of what you know and where you are. But the goal, I imagine, is to get to **CONSUMMATE LOVE**, which involves all three components. To feel a passionate desire to move, to be committed, and to know and build a culture with yourself!

Yes, I know, when we talk about love, we are almost always directing it toward some BooThang you are meant to be chasing or having. But you are the BooThang here! Loving *you* is the goal.

Love, to me, is like physics. "Energy cannot be created or destroyed; it can only be changed from one form to another." Einstein said this. For me, love can be transferred from person to person, from the you of the past to the you of the present, and helps to develop the you yet to come. Love is an alignment of energy that can create change as our understanding of love and self evolves and grows. So basically, as we *commit* to being *passionately* moved toward deeper *intimacy* with self, we have more *consummate* love with and for ourselves.

The point Schiraldi is trying to make is that you have to love on yourself. I am saying "love on" and not just "love" because love requires *action*. This means that—as a delightful woman once said in one of my weekly virtual community meetings called "In My Black Feelings"—how we care for ourselves, how we treat our bodies, and how we give to ourselves becomes a measuring stick for how we show ourselves love. (And this measure includes what we say to ourselves, too, because let's be real, some of us say some really f'ed up things to ourselves that we would never say to someone else.)

There is no single correct way to show ourselves love or care, despite what some might think. Even the things that look unhelpful can still offer us some help, some movement, and even some comfort, up to a point.

What we do is entirely adaptive. When it no longer works for where we are going or what we want for ourselves in the next phase, we have to love on ourselves differently, which may require undoing what was once done or learning to show ourselves love in a whole new way.

✍ JOURNAL WORK

Do you love yourself? What kind of love are you in, for the most part, right now? How do you know?

GROWING

The idea of growing is what we tend to be hyperobsessed with. We want to grow into the biggest and best versions of ourselves through learning, earning, and doing. The problem is that we think we can create love and worth in ourselves through all this learning, earning, and doing. But it doesn't work like that. The worth is meant to be unconditional, and the loving is meant to be an action-based embodiment of that worth.

You use unconditional worth and loving acts to boost your growth. Because when you have unconditional worth, you are more willing to try things. Because when you love on yourself, you take care of yourself in radical ways, including letting folk go from your life, and doing what you can toward your growth. This is why growing comes last on the list, because you cannot grow your way into loving yourself. You cannot grow your way into unconditional worth. It's innate, which means what we need to do is dust off the BS that has gotten in the way, not move toward it like a target.

And even though that's not how it works, people certainly have tried to do it that way. You may have tried, too. You may have tried to earn love with how you behave and found that when you stopped or couldn't continue the behavior, the so-called "love" you were experiencing from others, or even from yourself, went away.

☕ TEA TIME

Is it tea time already? Go grab a cup and come back. Here is some of my tea: I was def a person who thought you could behave and earn your way into self-esteem. I have been in that mindset of *if I could just get good grades* or *if I could just get the nice clothes,* then people would like me, I would like me, and it would help others to see and enjoy my company. I thought that if I got a romantic partner, I would be seen as valuable and worthy. I thought that if I could figure out how to have lighter skin, straighter hair, a smaller nose, a bigger ass, and be smart but not too smart, I would be the worthiest person on the planet. So, I tried to people-please my way into self-esteem. Being what people wanted me to be, hearing them say nice things, and even going after the degrees my parents wanted (doctor, lawyer, engineer). I was so busy chasing this clout that I never really got into the business of seeing my worth outside of what I could do for others. I never loved on myself—more like I would push myself to the breaking point and call it perseverance or discipline. I was trying to earn educational accolades, partners, friends, and beauty as a road toward loving myself and proving my worth. But that was never going to work. It couldn't work because if you fail a class, if you lose the partner, if your friends abandon you, or if your beauty fades, then you have nothing and return to nothing. Except that you are already someone of worth, unconditionally. Bay-bee, let me tell you: even when I was just *starting* to get there, things changed. I disappointed my parents, showed up more as myself, was more likely to say what I wanted from a romantic interest, found myself with friends I actually vibed with, and started seeing my beauty as simply different than what was popular.

We have a desire to grow, and many of us want to be the undisputed best. Because being the best would prove our worth and that we are well loved. But while we may grow in doing something and it could be awesome, we may never be the undisputed best. I mean, think about it, even Beyoncé, Michael Jackson, and Michael Jordan aren't undisputed as the best. It is very much disputed. People will tell you all day who they think are better singers, performers, and players on the court. People will pit folk against each other. And then there are those annoying posts on social media always asking you to choose from a list of artists which one has to go (along with their entire body of work). The comments always vary, because we all have a different idea and connection to each of the options. We all grew differently to appreciate different things. If Beyoncé, Michael Jackson, or Michael Jordan only did what they did for the accolades and used it as a way to like themselves and to prove their worth, they would be at the mercy of their critics, not their fans. They would be trying to find ways to appease the folk who do dispute what they do and how great they are. They would be seeking out ways to make people like them through the ceaseless, merciless pursuit of what they are good at while never exploring anything new. Not new sounds, not new business ventures. Nothing.

The point of all this is that you cannot buy, learn, or earn your way to loving yourself nor can you buy, learn, or earn your way to having worth. And while I personally may not agree with much, I definitely agree with that. You *can* be the best you, and damn if I don't wanna see that!

Knowing the components and steps to growing self-esteem, to healing it, is important. But we couldn't start here when you have to know what your components are first. No one chooses it except for you. And while it can seem counterintuitive, I wanted to include this section for a couple of reasons.

1. There isn't much that is new under the sun. Which means that if I am gonna give you the real-real, I have to take my ego and wanting to be the most right out of the equation.

2. I agree that you have to know you are a person of worth, practice and "perfect" the processes of showing yourself admiration, care, affection, etc., so that when you love on others you do so from a full cup—not by emptying what you have for yourself into others, nor requiring that they empty themselves in order to love on you— since they can never fill your self-love cup for you. They can only show you how they love you, and you can use it as an example of building love up in and for yourself.

Now, let's talk about hierarchies!

MASLOW'S HIERARCHY OF NEEDS

If you have ever taken a Psych 101 course, then you probably ran across a man named Abraham Maslow and his hierarchy of needs. While not necessarily the norm, when I think about self-esteem and what makes it what it is and how to achieve it, I think about this. Maslow's hierarchy of needs dictates that human needs exist within a hierarchy, where the basic survival needs are toward the bottom, and the need for self-actualization is toward the top. The idea is that, like a video game, when you beat one level, you get to level up until you finally reach self-actualization—your full potential. Take a moment to look at my sexy pic!

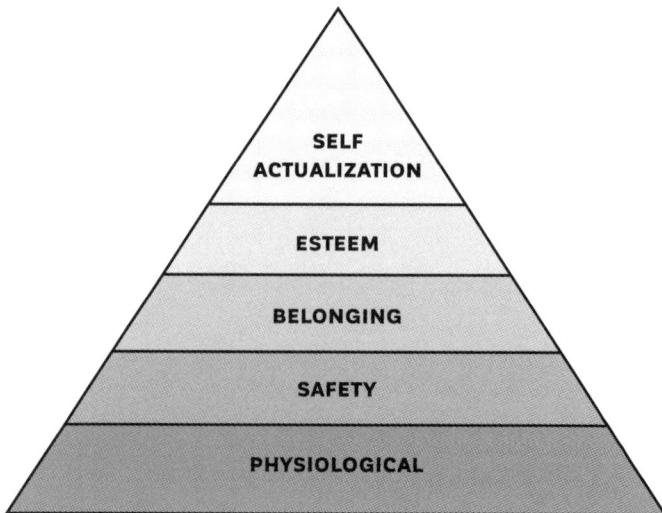

The needs on the hierarchy are as follows:

PHYSIOLOGICAL NEEDS. Air, water, food, shelter, sleep, clothing, sex, etc. These are physiological drives, as in your body is driving you to do the things that will help you stay alive.

SAFETY NEEDS. This includes physical and psychological safety. So, making sure your body is safe from harm, that you have the resources to continue that feeling of safety, including having a job, a place to lay your head, access to health-based resources, that type of stuff.

BELONGING. On this level, we are talking about having intimate relationships (intimacy and sex are not synonymous). These relationships could be with friends or family, or just feeling like you are connected in community. This can further enhance safety because when you have people, or when people have you, it can add to a feeling of safety, whether it's emotional or physical, or both.

ESTEEM. Were you waiting for it? Esteem here covers not only how we feel about ourselves but also the idea of respect, what our status is when we are alone and in community with others, recognition, strength, our personal security, employment, having resources, health, and property.

SELF-ACTUALIZATION. This is the top-top. It's the desire and ability to be all you can be…like the army slogan once said. At this point you are potenched.

How is this even applied to self-esteem?

Self-actualization is the goal, and self-esteem is required to achieve it. And honestly, isn't that why some of us want self-esteem? So we can feel better about ourselves and open the door to meeting our full potential?

If we leave Maslow's hierarchy of needs as-is, then we are in trouble. It basically says you have to earn your way to self-esteem and self-actualization, which is kind of fucked up. Think about it: one only has to look at history minutely to see that Black folk often live in food deserts and cannot trust the healthcare system nor the water from the tap. We only have to look at historical figures and watch the news to also understand that safety in Black bodies is far from guaranteed, and we can see clearly that they still consider us—the members of the global majority—to be a minority destined for marginalization, so there is a lack of the sense of belonging wholly. So, the needs that precede esteem are hardly met at the best of times. And here you are with the audacity of also being a Black woman. Um...yikes!

You might be reading and asking, "Well, then why the hell would you tell me about this?" I am telling you about Maslow's hierarchy because it still has merit to help us understand what else is in self-esteem. But what if I told you it was upside down? When perspectives shift and we add a little context, we can rock our own worlds!

Maslow didn't get this idea on his own; he studied the Blackfoot people, an indigenous population who were uprooted and placed on reservations in what is now known as Alberta,

Canada, and Montana, U.S.[5] The Blackfoot people's way of viewing this hierarchy would have self-actualization at the bottom. Though it should be noted that neither they nor Maslow ever actually put their concept into the triangle/pyramid form. The Blackfoot folk believed that you came into the world *already* self-actualized and that you simply lived up to the self-actualization through your actions within the community structure. A community structure that would band together to ensure that physiological needs were met, that the community enjoyed a sense of safety and belonging and had the respect of the others in the community. Sound familiar? To me, it sounds like how we treat babies. We see all their potential and simply make room for them. But then age, capitalism, sexism, racism, etc., get in the way and move actualization to the top shelf; then they tell you that you have to earn what should have been (and was) freely given. The Blackfoot people, they moved from a community standpoint. The community has responsibility and a role to play in each community member being all they can be. Maslow, as an American white man, however, was likely informed from an individualistic capitalist standpoint. So, you have to prove yourself worthy and earn the right to live to your potential.

My point is that Maslow's hierarchy of needs, when done the Blackfoot way, means that you require community to reach your full potential; you can't reach it on your own. And here you thought I told you to grab a friend to read this book with because I was blowing smoke up your ass. Nah. I also said it because there is a quote that says, "If you want to go fast, go alone. If you want to go far, go together." Getting far into self-esteem is a team sport.

Here we are, at the end of this chapter. I know it's pretty heavy shit. But the point is this: context matters when we talk about self-esteem, because the components change according to the different people who are choosing them. What makes up self-esteem is up to you, but we also have to know that what we choose and how we choose it can lead us to a type of self-esteem that is not for us, nor is it sustainable for what we may ultimately want to do. I sincerely hope that you will be honest with yourself about where on the spectrum you are and in which situations that changes for you. You wouldn't be lying to anyone but you about you. **shrug**

If you should decide that a life of liking and maybe even of loving yourself is what you want, I want to be clear that it will not be without outcomes that are both positive and negative. Some folk will want to put you "in your place," and others will laud you for your authenticity and the way you let your light shine. You have to choose for yourself which route you will take.

CHAPTER 3

Do You VALUE Self-Esteem?

Black women spend a lot of time waiting. We wait for permission to live our lives to the fullest. We wait for parents to tell us that we're allowed to go for the thing that we want. We wait for partners to say that they support us. We wait on jobs to give us promotions. We wait. We will spend a lifetime waiting, never pursuing the things that we desire because no one has given us permission. And when I say no one has given us permission, I mean *no one*! We have not even given ourselves permission to move forward. Are you familiar with the movie *Penelope,* the story of the little white girl with the pig nose? One thing I love about that movie is that at the end of the day, marriage to someone who was not worthy of her time, attention, or affection was not the route that she chose to go. She chose instead to run away to possibly live the rest of her life with her little piggy nose, alone.

What's more, she learned to love herself in the process. She gave *herself* permission to live her life. She was no longer in a holding pattern, waiting for her face to be fixed in order for her life to start. She chose to give value and credence to her self-esteem, which she was not taught to value by her family. She was taught to seek and value the male gaze, external validation, and conventional beauty, much like many of us have been taught. She was taught that she would be valuable as soon as she was married. She chose to value herself and have self-esteem despite her family (or her face).

✍ JOURNAL WORK

With this in mind, here are my questions to you:

1. In what areas of your life are you in a holding pattern? Have you given yourself permission to stop living your life in a holding pattern? How?
2. Have you given yourself permission to have self-esteem, not just internally, but to live a life as someone with self-esteem, outwardly?
3. Do you even value self-esteem? How do you know?

What Are Values, Anyway?

As a therapist, I have heard some truly weird shit. But nothing takes the cake more than an email from a colleague to a group of therapists asking, "Who charges the most for therapy?" while telling us that we can't charge less than $250. You see, they had a client who wanted *the best* therapist they could find in their geographical state. It was weird to see therapists respond to this email with their prices, hoping that they won. Who doesn't want to be paid more? *I didn't compete. I wasn't licensed in the state, but I think I couldda won...well, almost!*

Now, you might be thinking, "Why was a client looking for the most expensive therapy?!?!" Well, she figured that if it cost more, then it's a better value. I, too, have fallen into this trap. I don't want the most expensive, and I don't want the least expensive. The saying, "You get what you pay for," rings loud as hell in my head when I am searching for deals. I never wanted to be cheated out of good value.

Now, I don't know about you, but one of the first ever definitions of *value* that I had was monetary value. If I had to buy it with money, then it had value. How much value something had was almost always related to how much it cost. This could be why so many people want a hookup. It means the thing you are hooking them up with has value, but they get to pay less than that value. Isn't that why so many of us fall in love with Marshalls or the value pack of toilet paper from Costco? We feel like we are cheating the system by getting more monetary value for less!

Basically, values guide what we feel, think, and how we behave. Values tell us what is important, desirable, useful, or worth our while. Values become the *why* behind what we think, say, and do.

✐ *JOURNAL WORK*

VALUES

Grab a piece of paper and make two columns, labeled "Values" and "Impacts." Under the "Values" column, list your top five values. Take a moment to consider each of these values thoughtfully. Then, in the "Impacts" column, write about how each of these values have impacted your emotions, thoughts, and behaviors.

The Role Values Play in Self-Esteem

Looking at the definition of *values*, I hope you can already see a hazy picture of where I am going. The point here is that how we have been taught to value self-esteem is based on "value relative to others." That means you may often value yourself according to what value you *think* you offer to others, which then confirms or denies your worth, or value. How do we know this? We know this because in the idea of self-concept by Carl Rogers, he talks about how if parents/caregivers heap praise and give unconditional positive regard, it can give us a sense of self-concept or self-esteem, which is then congruent with what our experiences are with others. Basically, we feel good about ourselves because other people confirm that we are good. On the other hand, if caregivers make love and/or acceptance conditional on behavior, grades, etc., then instead of showing up as ourselves, we hide our "bad" selves and undesirable behaviors, so we can be loved by our family (i.e., masking, though we tend to call it *code switching*). The thing is, we don't just stay within our families of origin. Our sense of self-esteem will fluctuate as we leave our homes of origin and go into the world. As a result of this, we often try to make ourselves more valuable to the people who are around us by mimicking their values. We wait on them to dub us as worthy, lovable, and valuable. From schools, to jobs, to friends and partners, they have to tell us that we are worthy of getting in, of being there for, and of love. They join the family of origin as a function of telling us our worth based on our value relative and in comparison to them. The problem is people who aggrandize themselves to give or not give permission for you to live *your* life, knowingly or unknowingly, are often looking out for *their own* best interest, not yours. Living their best life often includes having you play the role they have assigned you (i.e., family structure) to keep the routine of their life. Let's go back to *Penelope* as an example. Her mom ultimately gave her values with set expectations of her behavior. Mom wanted to avoid being embarrassed, creating the need for Penelope to be a recluse in order to satisfy her mom's value of conventional beauty. Also, by extension of her mother's values, she needed to seek out blue-blooded men as potential husbands in order to fix her face and validate both her (Penelope's) worth as a person with a pig nose and, by extension, her mother, for birthing a person with a pig nose. A recipe for low self-esteem.

This basically shows how we are not usually taught to see self-esteem as a real value, and we are not taught to see ourselves as valuable outside of what we can do for others. Caregivers give us value based on what we do for them or how we follow their rules and demonstrate/reflect their values back to them. Even if you don't get it there, this message is in other structures. Schools value students who follow their rules and demonstrate/reflect their values back to them. Same goes for team sports, jobs, and other organized spaces. If we are not careful, we recapitulate family-like structures in the various spaces encountered.

DIAGRAM A: TRIANGULATION/SELF ESTEEM

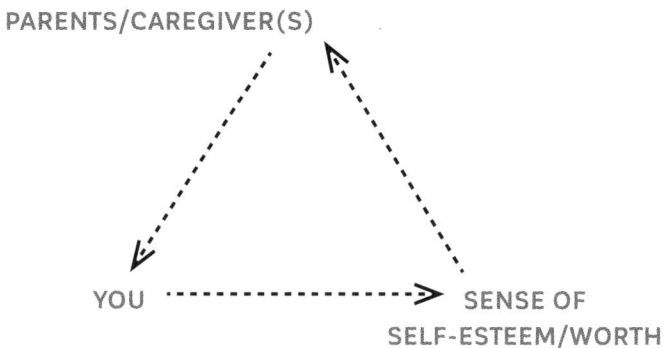

PARENTS/CAREGIVER(S)

YOU ·······················> **SENSE OF SELF-ESTEEM/WORTH**

Starting with you, the sense of self-esteem may feel separate as it is filtered through the dominant structure of the household (parent/caregiver[s]), before returning to you to give you a sense of self.

Now seems as good a time as any to talk more about family structure and triangulation. Argentinian therapist Salvador Minuchin's family structure "refers to the way a family is organized" into systems, regulated by boundaries, which creates patterns of interaction that require everyone to play their roles relative to the other people in the structure.[1] There goes that phrase again, *relative to others*. You may have heard that you should "stay in a child's place" growing up. Your family structure would have given an idea of what a child's place was meant to be. However, we all have roles in various structures, even aside from family of origin. When we don't play the role, we can create conflict in the structure; then triangulation can come into play.

Triangulation is defined by American psychiatrist Murray Bowen as a way to "detour conflict between two people by involving a third person, stabilizing the relationship between the original pair." Look y'all, I am using *people* loosely. I am using it because we are talking about systems and structures that involve people and, thus, relationships. Furthermore, the third person doesn't have to be a person; it can just be a stabilizing agent, applied or removed. *Remember when I told y'all that I think all these theories are just pieces of the whole? This is that pluriverse phenomena, for me. So just go with it.* When we play our role in our family and other systems/structures, there is a sense of homeostasis. The status quo is maintained. However, when we shirk the system, we upset the balance, and often a third party or thing is brought in to triangulate and bring order back. Meaning, we can get triangulated back to "our place" to help maintain the structures and bring relative homeostasis.

♨ *TEA TIME*

So, allow me to spill my own tea. In my family of origin, I have my parents and three younger sisters. I am the eldest Naija girl. This means that I have a predetermined role by my parents as to what I am supposed to do and who I am to be as the eldest. My role in the family structure was to lead, almost like a third parent (yeah, I was definitely a parentified child). My job is to set an example for my sisters by living in such a way that doesn't bring anyone (read: my parents) shame. For anyone who is also a first-gen kid, you may have heard that you must live your life to be a doctor, lawyer, or engineer. Anything less and they may be looking at you with some serious side-eye. I was on track for all of that. I was doing as I should—bringing home decent grades and properly hiding my "bad behavior." In leaving high school, becoming a lawyer was the original goal, but at the end of high school, I changed my plan to study psychology. It excited me.

Anyway, my parents rolled with it because I would be "a doctor of the psychology," thereby meeting the value and standard of behavior. In learning more about myself and my comfort though, I realized I wanted to be a sex therapist, and I didn't really have a desire to be a doctor of anything but sex. Enter, the problem: I was moving against the values of the family structure. I upset the homeostasis because I was outside of my role in the family structure. Can a sex therapist be an example to younger siblings? Does this career choice not bring shame to the family, especially in talking about a taboo subject?

Anyway, triangulation came into play with some very tough conversations, which hurt my feelings, but then a boon: my mom was onboard! However, I was, in some ways, turned away for not being within the structure by my father. This led to years of comments about my studies, or no questions at all. I was still somewhat supported, but

I wasn't *seen*. My father, and some other folk, needed to have some semblance of order in the structure, so I became the thing you didn't talk about. Their mental defense mechanisms were triggered, and instead of outward hostility, which proved ineffective in changing my will, I was disregarded and seen as something shameful.

(Change came slow for some of my folk, but it did come. My dad is the first one to brag now. It could have to do with the PhD in sexuality, or it could have to do with learning more about what a sex therapist actually does and seeing its value. Hm...maybe it's somewhere in the middle.)

The point is, when you become more in alignment with your own core values, and your sense of self-worth and -esteem are not filtered through the dominant structure of your family/caregivers, you can upset the balance if your behaviors are no longer in alignment with their expectations. It can lead to stern talks, ridicule, being disowned—all of which is done to triangulate you back into position and ease the structure back to a sense of homeostasis. The thing we forget is that while you are being triangulated to maintain the structure of your family, your family is not immune from the ways they are also triangulated into the system of the dominant American culture. Their self-esteem and sense of self are filtered through the white supremacist dominant and delusional American culture, and in their trying to simultaneously protect you from and meet the expectations of the culture, and in their pursuit to also secure their self-esteem and -worth, the intergenerational cycle of harm begins. Let's go back to *Penelope* real quick. The mom is triangulated into a system where she and her self-esteem are separated and filtered through the dominant cultural structure(s) (Diagram B).

DIAGRAM B: TRIANGULATION/SELF-ESTEEM

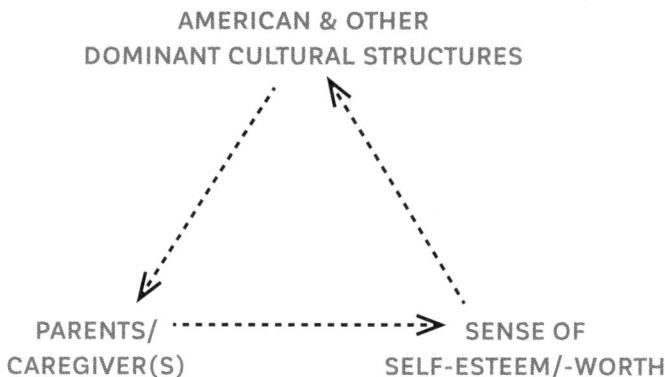

**AMERICAN & OTHER
DOMINANT CULTURAL STRUCTURES**

**PARENTS/
CAREGIVER(S)** - - - - - - - - - - - - -> **SENSE OF
SELF-ESTEEM/-WORTH**

Her sense of self-esteem and values are filtered through the dominant culture, so she behaves in ways that reflect their values of beauty and wealth as a way to have/maintain a sense of power. She is only giving to her child what she has been taught to value: a way to secure herself with a husband, and thus prove herself an asset in the structure (Diagram C). Her child is the one who disrupts the system, breaking the chain of intergenerational harm by choosing herself. Securing her self-esteem becomes a show of claiming her power, which ironically, allows her entry into the very structures of power which value it. Sigh.

DIAGRAM C: TRIANGULATION/SELF-ESTEEM

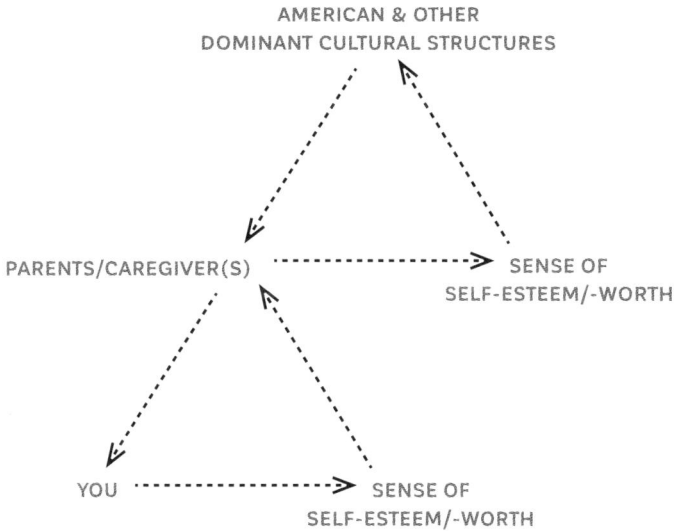

AMERICAN & OTHER
DOMINANT CULTURAL STRUCTURES

PARENTS/CAREGIVER(S) - - - - - - - - - - - - -> SENSE OF
SELF-ESTEEM/-WORTH

YOU - - - - - - - - - -> SENSE OF
SELF-ESTEEM/-WORTH

Self-esteem can't truly be valued by dominant culture on its own, because it often means that the structure can be waylaid by folk who don't share the same core values and go their own way. Unless their way still includes one of the more important penchants of the structure, namely capitalism. And we have already said cultures and subcultures find various things useful and will see the value relative to its importance and the desirability in that given culture. Yes, values from one culture to the next can contradict each other. For example, on one side of things you have Scruff McGruff, the Crime Dog, relaying his value for order by asking you to take a bite out of crime by reporting what you see. However, I don't know about you, but when I was growing up my subculture said, "Snitches get stitches." This is just one example of how a culture's values can contradict another's, where power and dominance play a role. With dominant culture and subcultures constantly at play, being what each structure wants you to be (playing your role) can be fraught with pitfalls leading to anxiety and a feeling of not being adequate at navigating (also known as threats to your self-esteem). Though many a Black person prides themself on their ability to code switch given their location and who is present, there is still a strain. Let's talk more about dominant cultural values.

American Values

One of the main dominant cultures that will be present throughout this book is American culture. The *white* in *American values* is silent. I wasn't sure if you heard it. Let's use the Johari window to talk about American values and how this is the soil in which we are to plant our self-esteem. Or to put it another way, this is the CONTEXT.

Things to note before we get started: If you read the introduction (and I hope you did), then you know that I am about to be biased as hell. You also know there is no such thing as objectivity where people are concerned. We are always inclined to side with someone, even if it's just that you are secretly (or out loud) rooting for the Black family when you watch *Family Feud*. We don't really hold neutrality that well because our experiences inform who we are and how we choose to move. As such, you should know that my view of America's window is based on my personal experience. This is my view as a dark-skinned, kinky-haired, Black, Nigerian-American woman therapist and as a person who reads a lot and talks to a lot of people. The person that you are will also interact with my view. It can ring true, false, or somewhere in between. Feel me? Alright, here we go.

AMERICA'S WINDOW

PUBLIC: It would seem to me that the public values are freedom, opportunity, and achievement. To talk about the public face of America, the perspective of the immigrant, like my parents, who only really saw America on TV or heard about its greatness from the media and other sources, is a great place to start. My parents, like much of the world, were taught that America is the land of freedom and opportunity, where anyone who works hard can achieve their wildest dreams. There is this sense of having the ultimate makeover, America at the helm, to help you go from rags to riches, as it were, as long as you trust the process and do your part (i.e., work hard). In pulling yourself up, fashioned by American individualism, you can have the American dream! The American dream includes a two-level home, two and a half children (How exactly do you have a half of a child?), a dog (preferably a golden retriever), and a white picket fence. Of course this is also achieved in a heterosexual, monogamous marriage that reflects the traditional values of a breadwinning father and a caretaking mother (who may also work, but more as a hobby). When I think of the

American dream, it takes me back to watching TGIF as a kid. The line up included *Family Matters, Boy Meets World,* and *Step by Step.* Did you sing the intro in your head a little? That *Step by Step* family was the American dream...well, revised. The dream doesn't usually include a divorce, but with their large blended family, they spoke about the dream, right in the damn theme song! I could never quite put my finger on why, but that show always made me think about *Full House*: two and a half kids and a dog. While both of these shows fall shy of having the perfect American dream in romantic partnership, they certainly had it in real estate, kids, animals, and whiteness. Cuz isn't that the unspoken part of the American dream, that it's for white folk?

PRIVATE: Now, the private self of America values power, capitalism, and patriarchy, not necessarily in that order. As wholesome as the public face is, the inner workings and unspoken values are almost an underbelly. The wholesomeness of the American dream is built on stolen land and built by stolen and enslaved people. How can you pull yourself up by your bootstraps when you are actually stealing shit from other people? This goes to show the often-contradictory nature of how we name our values and how we live them. What's funny is that none of this feels very private, especially not lately. Our shenanigans are more and more on display. In "private," we value having power, money, and a penis, while trying to maintain the good-guy public facade about anyone having opportunity and freedom to achieve. When, really, the story is that the folk who have the freedom and opportunity to really achieve are white men, especially if they have Daddy giving them a "small" loan of anything from a couple hundred thousand to a million dollars.

The problem is our valuing of rich white men is very visible, from corporations to Hollywood and our government. People like to see businesses and governments led by men, who are thought of as being more level-headed, logical, and having a right to lead that was granted to them by God, which also makes even religion toe the line of valuing patriarchy over all else. Hell, don't we also like our movies with a heavy dose of male lead? However, it is almost always explained as a simple happenstance derived from the natural order of men leading and women supporting and following behind. Thus affirming the power of men and their right to rule by way of patriarchy. Men with money are even further chosen by God, as they have now shown their mental prowess in how they have been able to maintain their households and businesses by way of their wallets. So, capitalism, and who has the bigger bank account, also becomes synonymous with power and men. Rich men, then, are the ones who have the power to control not only the government at large, which is a huge visual cue because they are seen as being more capable of leading, but they have control of women right down to our reproductive rights—you know, shit that don't make no sense.

Coming off politics and moving into Hollywood and corporations, in the media and in movies there has been some research, inspired by the joke of the Bechdel-Wallace Test, , that shows men tend to have more speaking lines than women.[2] Additionally, we already know that Hollywood, like the rest of the country, has a pay gap problem. None of this stuff is new, none of this stuff is surprising, and all of this stuff is regular. Women get paid eighty cents to a man's dollar.[3] We also know that women only account for less than six percent of Global 500 CEOs, according to Fortune. The valuing of capitalism, patriarchy, and power is well established and seen but only as a happenstance of who is just more fit to naturally lead, as opposed to being a visual and acted-out cue of American values.[4]

BLIND: Moving on to the blind self, where the values of whiteness and appearances live. I am not going to spend too much time here. The point is this, we have a "hidden" way of constantly valuing and centering whiteness without ever really needing to name it. Go google something to do with almost any subject and you will see things related to white folk as a default. You actually have to specify that you are looking for PoC or Black folk in order to get those results. If you look again at the previous section on private values, you will see that I kept talking about rich white men. Rich. *White*. Men. Because part of the caveat for the American dream is whiteness and maleness together. We value the rich and we value men, but that's only (or rather, especially) if you're white! Stats about women making eighty cents to a man's dollar is a *white* statistic! Black folk, women of color, and Black women actually make varying levels of more or less than that, with Black women usually just trailing! Yet, that's the stat folk love to use. Five percent of companies having a woman at the helm is an alarming statistic until you also remember that 1.2 percent are women of color!

Appearances, on the other hand, have already been (in)directly spoken about. America is all about the appearance of opportunity, freedom, and achievement, based in individualistic rhetoric. For some, namely the people who are at the center or just left of center of American values, it feels progressive, forward thinking, and inclusive. But for those on the margins, we see that America is much like a lot of other white people who have their blinders on and use emotional manipulation like a daily tool. These are people who would say they're not racist and do racist shit every day all day. America either fails to understand that it's mostly backward in favor of the rich white man and screws itself over in the process or knows but secretly doesn't desire change because, hello, identity crisis! Who is America if it doesn't uplift the (white) male mediocrity of folk who steal from others, while thinking themselves virtuous and more valuable? But I digress. Within the blind self is the division of thoughts, feelings, and behaviors. What you think, what you feel, and what you do are not as separate as folk think. And thus, we are not as effective at separating them as we would like to believe. America tries to show the world (public) progressive behaviors. Those thoughts however (private) still seep through in the outward behavior. Even worse, it doesn't really understand the emotions of fear and anxiety (blind) that motivate and inform the thoughts and behaviors.

UNKNOWN: Unknown.

What you see in America's Johari window may be the same, different, expanded, or contracted. Looking at the evidence, we see that women have been sidetracked while patriarchy is centered. We also know that Black people are marginalized and whiteness is centered. But where are Black women? The answer is that we are at the intersection of dealing with sexism *and* racism. Our intersection helps to support the machine, but it is a thankless, backbreaking job, with little to no benefit to us. Why? Because in this machine, our value relative to the dominant American culture steeped in whiteness and maleness, is minimal at best and nonexistent at worst, which can spell disaster for our self-esteem.

We know "actions speak louder than words." We are way more likely to imitate behavior than we are to listen to someone tell us not to do something that they are doing. The problem is caregivers and the larger system we are encased in don't value Black women. This means we can be mimicking and filtering our self-worth, -esteem, and -identity through these systems to our own detriment. It can lead to a feeling of emptiness even though we are heaped with praise by others for being strong in the face of it all. Living our lives with others' values at the center is a loss of power that we profoundly feel.

Our attempt to navigate it and succeed doesn't give us time to learn or know our core values, which are integral to our development and maintenance of self-esteem. Again, look at *Penelope*. She saw herself the way her mother saw her, as someone unacceptable, unlovable, on the margins, unworthy of self-esteem. Knowing and understanding the external structures allowed her (and will allow you) more space to see what has been impacting her while giving her a broader sense of control...a.k.a. power. Penelope's power was developed and honed by trying shit out, learning the various values others could hold, finding her tribe, and choosing herself. Knowing where the values around you lie, and knowing you are not a failure for having adhered to their poison for most of your life, helps you to claim your self-esteem as a value, directly, or indirectly, by living for yourself and not through others.

In an effort to help you feel more empowered, you have some values-based homework. Cuz like Maya said, and has been quoted already in this book: "When we know better, we do better."

✐ JOURNAL WORK

VALUES ORIGIN

For this homework, you will create your own Johari window. Think about your public and private faces in life. In each win- dowpane, where do each of your values land? *Don't worry, you can add more than the top five I originally asked for.* Then think about where each of those values came from and how they have or have not been practiced. Are there values you want that are not present? Which ones? What would it look like to live by those values?

CHAPTER 4

What We Not Gon' Do!

Historically, books about self-esteem have not included the Black woman's experience. We already know this, at the very least, because I've said it in this book. Those books make it seem like self-esteem is a universal concept that applies to everyone equally, but that's only because they default to white. And when it comes to talking about self-esteem among Black people, we default to light. Yes, we default to the light-skinned girl being the one who automatically gets to have expressed self-esteem, while everyone else has to prove themselves as worthy, usually through proximity to whiteness or desirability. Sounds familiar, right?

What we not gon' do is ignore colorism as a part of who gets to express self-esteem. What we not gon' do is ignore the role that white and male supremacy play in the pick-me politics that women use. Nor will we pretend that being a victim of circumstance means that there is something wrong with *you* rather than the *system* you were born into. So, as my sister would say: "Buckle up, buttercup." We got work to do.

Tropes of Black Womanhood

In the world of bestowed tropes, there are none more played out for Black women than the tropes of the Mammy, the Jezebel, and the Sapphire—all of which are tied into the white gaze's interpretation of Black womanhood. And we wouldn't have to work too hard to find examples of these tropes in popular media and culture.

Now, not everyone is familiar with these tropes, so I am going to explain them.

THE MAMMY is often described as the fat, dark-skinned, kinky-haired woman who is all too happy to serve the white families. She is happy with her lot in life and has no ambition to see change, just to serve and be of help to the white folk to whom she is tied. She is also seen as sexually undesirable. Someone who no one would want to have sex with. In this section, we are gonna leave some of her sexuality out, but we are gonna get into what it means for self-esteem. The point is that the Mammy is disempowered because she is fat, and, as a society, we have decided that fat bodies should not exist (read: genocide) because we believe that they are unhealthy (as though people owe you health or as though the size of a body is indicative of health, but I digress). The point here is that she is disempowered because she is dark, and kinky, and fat. The idea being that she is not worthy of attention, affection, or love until she loses the weight and gets a weave. Now while she can't do much about her dark skin, she can control her weight and do something about her hair. If she is bold, she can also quietly erase the darkness of her skin with bleaching creams. In controlling herself, she would gain control and a sense of desire that would grant her permission to like herself.

We have to note that we don't always see the Mammy portrayed in the exact same way—as the dark fat kinky-haired woman. Often, something is changed. They will change her hair, or they will make her a person interested in losing weight (or remove weight altogether as a factor), or we will see light-skinned fat Black women. But the idea here is that something has to give in order to make her into something/someone that is more worthy, though she may still serve as the comic relief.

THE SAPPHIRE is described as brown skinned. Someone who might be halfway desirable if not for her mouth and power to emasculate others. Because the Sapphire is so emasculating and rubs against male supremacy in the wrong way, she is often met with violence from folk who would like to put her in her place. She is called a "bitch." She is not considered pretty enough to be that mean. It's about calling out her audacity and moving her to where they want her to be.

THE JEZEBEL is characterized by her light skin, wavy hair, and Eurocentric-leaning features. The Jezebel's—labeled as such because men's power is defined by their ability to get the best women and to fuck those women—power lies in the fact that men want to fuck her and use her as a trophy. She is desirable, but she's still not a person. However, she is a person with power *because* she is desirable. She's wifey material. And because she's desirable and wifey material, she elevates the status of the men who desire *and are able to* get her. She is valued in how she walks the line in ambiguousness, because she is not viewed as being fully Black, even if she is. She gets to use the power of her allure as a foundation for her sense of self-esteem. But that self-esteem still doesn't belong to her; it's bestowed by others because of what she looks like, not because of who she is.

These tropes can make a Black girl feel hella one-dimensional. And the thing is, they still make themselves known in how we have and express our self-esteem. They have a role in how we feel about ourselves, the experiences we have had, and the way we carry ourselves.

"You're Acting Light Skinned"

In the world of Black girls, it's the light-skinned ones who get to have expressed self-esteem. When I say *expressed* I mean that their self-esteem gets to have words and actions that others hear and see and are even likely to accept. We know it's true because it comes up in phrases like "You're acting light skinned," particularly when directed at a dark-skinned person—because the notion here is that you are not pretty and privileged enough to have expressed self-esteem.

What does it mean to be acting light skinned? Well, when that one is thrown around among women (and femmes especially), we are talking about conventionally (the convention being white supremacy) beautiful women supposedly behaving like they are better or cuter than other high-maintenance, superior, picky, "extra," uppity, feminine, and overall better than dark-skinned women. When a man/masculine person is told they are acting light skinned, it carries the same definition, but there is an emphasis on the feminine/effeminate manner of that person, though not in a favorable manner.

Let's get into the expressed self-esteem part of it. A few ways that we might express self-esteem are in being more assertive with our language, having boundaries that we also tell folk about, experiencing and expecting secure relationships, being more congruent in what you say and what you do (walking the walk and talking the talk). Basically, behaving the way we think someone with high self-esteem might behave. Some may call it *main character syndrome*.[1]

And there is *nothing* wrong with that! There is nothing wrong with being assertive, having boundaries, sharing your thoughts or ideas, feeling secure in your relationships or any of that. The problem is that some women (i.e., dark-skinned women) do not have the same access to it because they don't have pretty privilege. *Pretty privilege* is the concept that more-attractive people receive unearned benefits in society simply for being, well, pretty.

When the phrase "You're acting light skinned" is thrown out, even jokingly, it is usually an explanation and/or an admonishment of someone's behavior. For light-skinned girls, it can be an explanation that they are expected to behave a certain way and their behavior might be simultaneously admired while being annoying. But make no mistake, it is also thrown out as a warning that a dark-skinned someone is "acting above their station." Yes, I said *station*. This is a way light-skinned women are told they are doing too much, while also being a way to tell darker-skinned women that they are not pretty enough to be doing that much.

Dark-skinned girls are loud, masculine, disrespectful, and ugly. Light-skinned girls are feminine, beautiful, docile, and desirable. The horn and halo effects in practice. The *halo effect* is a psychology term used to describe a condition in which a positive attribute is assigned to a group of people or a single person, so we then go beyond that to say they must be good overall due to that one positive attribute. The opposite is also true: if we assign a negative attribute to something, we will demonize it—the *horn effect*. Dark-skinned people, especially dark skinned women, are often demonized, where light-skinned people, especially light-skinned women, are often made out to be good. We will come back to more of this soon. But first, let's get into some tropes.

Casting Call!

In Chapter 3, I talked about the roles we have in our families and how when we change our roles, we also change our families. Sometimes the family members come willingly into new territory, but a lot of times, they go kicking and screaming and work hard to drag us back to the role they have needed us to play. This is true for society at large. We have all been cast into a certain role.

WHITE SUPREMACY PRODUCING...

White men have been self-cast as the pinnacle of our society, a position reinforced through worldwide violence and systemic oppression. They are "good," "fair," "smart," and "chosen by God to lead." White women are made, in this delusion, to support white men by holding them up, being their ear, cleaning up their messes, and producing their progeny. They are protected and valued by white men, though their role is a subordinate one. Now, I know you can see where we are going. Because the dead opposite of the white light of "goodness" is the dark depths, blackness. Black people as a whole are cast as being the opposite of whatever white is supposed to be. We are considered to be "bad," "dark," "stupid," and "created by God to serve." Now, hopefully you know that's bullshit. However, if we are being really real, then we also know that even if we don't believe it, too many of us are still caught up in these tropes and roles.

MALE SUPREMACY REQUESTS...

When you think about what male supremacy requests, it often requests our objectification. It requires us to soothe and calm. To love and be a soft landing. It requires us to be sexual receptacles and fodder for entertainment. Now there isn't anything wrong with doing any of that if it brings you pleasure. But no one wants to be defined by what white folk want or by what masculine people want.

The problem with these definitions is that they have been poured into us since we were young. Some of us choose to fight them and define ourselves in opposition to them, and some of us acquiesce and choose to define ourselves by being the best at what is being requested.

But what we not gon' do is pretend that going with it or being oppositional is the same thing as defining yourself *for* yourself. Defining yourself within or to be opposite of still means they got to trigger a move in you to even make a choice. Defining yourself requires thought, work, and, yes, some healing.

Now some would say that you can't make any decisions outside of social and structural power because of its pervasive presence—and for the most part, I agree. It is very difficult to know who you would be and how you would show up if supremacy culture, as we know it, wasn't so very baked into our every day.

So, before we really get started, I invite you to sit and imagine.

✐ JOURNAL WORK

Consider what life would have been like if you were not born into a world where, as Marvel Comic's villian-turned-hero Loki would say, we are "in a mad scramble for power, for identity." If you got to be a human being and didn't have to prove your worth. If people weren't considered better than another, but rather just folk who are equal in standing. If white supremacy, male supremacy, etc., weren't a thing. If capitalism wasn't a dogged pursuit to prove oneself better than another. If all your basic needs were more than adequately met, and you had no fear of racism, sexism, homophobia, transphobia, ableism, etc. What would you be doing? What life would you be living? What would you desire for yourself?

If you are anything like me, this is a difficult exercise. One, because the dream space has been denied to us by way of hustle-and-grind culture, which requires our ceaseless labor. Secondly, because it's hard to imagine something you have not seen or experienced. But when I tried hard-hard, I saw an unraveling. My whole world as I knew it changed. In pulling one thread, I saw a bit more of how it was intertwined with others. I imagine I would have been a dancer, because in my world where supremacy culture doesn't exist, parents also simply allow a child to be who and what they are. So, I would have danced. I would likely have still fallen in love with psychology, but I would have seen movement as the thing to bring us in, to stop us being disembodied. But then, I figured, without supremacy, would there have been colonialism as we know it? So, then I considered, would my parents have moved across the world at all? Would the story of Jesus have been strong in Yorubaland? If Khemet wasn't destroyed nor ancient Egypt, what would have existed across Africa? Without human supremacy what species of animals would still exist? How might we have built things that also help to sustain our planet versus fattening a few pockets? The world unraveled, but what I found was myself in love and joy and peace. I imagined myself living for my pleasure, connected with self and others. I saw myself never struggling with my skin tone, hair texture, facial features, or gender. I saw myself. And in seeing myself, I also saw, accepted, and appreciated others. I saw all kinds of bodies dressed and adorned in all kinds of ways and saw the world as being better and richer for it.

And while this world may not exist for you now, it doesn't mean you cannot cultivate it. But it means we cannot ignore, dismiss, or diminish the impacts that supremacy culture actually has on us. Some would tell us to forget about it, or tell us that thinking about and noting it means we are behaving in a victim's mentality. But what mentality does someone who has been harmed have? What mentality does a person who has been tricked or used as a sacrifice have? One where they note it? Where they are cautious? No, we do a good job of blaming the victim for remaining a victim while never giving any of that smoke to the people and systems that create victims in the first place. We forget that victims are often busy rebuilding the lives that were disrupted or that they are contemplating a way through, working on healing and being vigilant that they will not be in the same circumstance again. Does that sound like "no work" to you?

I am not asking you to be a victim; I am asking you to stop taking responsibility for other people's shit and calling it empowerment.

Critical-thinking questions here: Who defined what a victim is and noted what a victim mentality is? Who defined it? If history serves as a show of repeats, then we know the lion has called the sheep a victim while removing themselves from the equation.

What we not gon' do, though, is pretend that white and male supremacy have not helped to determine which Black girls and women get to have expressed self-esteem and then would not still punish them later for being "too uppity."

Identity Development and Self-Esteem

Here is the thing: dark-skinned girls are expected to have stable low self-esteem. We think there is nothing to shine on, so there is no reason to feel good. And while I have certainly seen that in my time as a therapist, I more often see the one with damaged self-esteem. We do the self-esteem assessment, and within it I ask my clients where they think their self-esteem is. They often report a low number on a scale of 0 to 100. However, in comparison to the assessment score, their estimation is low while the assessment of their self-esteem is higher. Damaged by the world around them which is constantly reconfirming that they are not pretty enough, valuable enough, or "the shit" enough to be "acting light skinned."

Light-skinned girls, on the other hand, are more likely to have fragile self-esteem, from what I see. Particularly when self-esteem is based on what they look like and not who they are as a person. This is the self-esteem that looks present and pretty on the outside but is damn near nonexistent on the inside. There is a constant seeking and needing of external validation that there is beauty and value—something that is reconfirmed in music ("I like a thick, long-haired, red bone"), shown as pinnacle desirable Black women in media, and something sought after and protected, particularly in Black communities. The validation-seeking is not just of being pretty and desirable, but it's also of being Black. Because if light-skinned girls have their Black cards revoked, then they may very quickly move to low stable self-esteem because they would either be compared to only other biracial and light-skinned Black women, or they would be lumped in with white women and would never be considered white enough. White people will not give them that edge or the privileges that would come with it. Black people, on the other hand, will. So, there is almost an unconscious desire to be the intermediary class and be the highest of the low instead of the lowest of the high.

The point of this chapter is this: in the world of self-esteem healing, we don't get to call on community and dismiss community damage. We don't get to call on so-called independence and forget we are an interdependent species in a great ecosystem of life. Knowing how to fix something comes with knowing the elements that add to its wrongness.

What we not gon' do is default to white, and we don't default to light either.

Other Sh*t We Not Gon' Do

Now this list is not necessarily going to be covered throughout the rest of this book. But sometimes knowing how we participate is half the battle. When you read this list, consider what you are already engaging in. Consider how you can try to be more conscious of it. Consider who in your crew you can recruit to help hold you accountable. Consider if you need to learn more about the phenomenon and set aside time dedicated to your research and reflection. And be sure to check the resource section at the back of this book. It will list a few things you can use to continue your learning, growth, and facilitate change.

So, here are some of the things we not gon' do:

→ **Use borrowed views of ourselves.** Especially from people who don't like us. As Nikki Giovanni said, we have the wrong audience when we ask people who hate us if we are pretty.[2]

→ **Act like emotions, thoughts, and behaviors are all the same thing but with different names.** We are gonna work to understand how we feel, know what we think, and make choices for how we behave!

→ **See being a Black woman as the problem.** Being Black is glorious, delightful, fun. Being a woman can feel hella sensual and peaceful. Being a Black woman isn't the problem. The white supremacist and patriarchal delusions of seeing Black folk and women as inferior and being in need of control is the problem. Supremacy culture is what's terrifying, dangerous, and exhausting. Watch your words, love.

→ **Act like respectability politics will save us.** What we not gon' do is act like respectability politics are the route to happiness and safety. There are a few great people who were shot while they wore suits. Not to mention the mental health challenges that come with having to mask around those in positions of supposed power. So STAHP IT!

→ **Think that self-love is self-taught.** I said what I said. We are not gon' keep looking at people like they failed in life because they have not yet figured out self-esteem. How we feel about ourselves is often inherited and repeated behavior from those around us.

→ **Confuse the absence of pain with the presence of pleasure.** As we move into the healing, we are not gon' mistake not being in constant pain with finally living in pleasure. They are not the same.

→ **Code switching and masking**. Cuz you don't have to be

anyone but you. Besides, if we continue with masking and code switching, the people who are not us never build up their "tolerance" for our authenticity. But even if you are not yet in the space to show up like you, you can choose which elements to bring forward. Those of us who can show up will, and hopefully it will feel safer for you in time.

→ **Enact self-imposed time poverty to get out of feeling our feels.** This is where we tell ourselves that we don't have time, when we do. We are just avoiding our feelings. We use TV, social media, a sudden desire to clean the house, ANYTHING. Stop. Take ten minutes and just feel your feels. You deserve that self-consideration.

→ **Gaslight ourselves.** What we not gon' do is engage in self-gaslighting, telling ourselves things like, "You're just being dramatic." Your pain, however it shows up, is worthy of acknowledgment and room. We aren't calling it dramatic. Especially not when you prolly been holding it in for a good long-assed time.

I am sure there are other things we not gon' do, but I would like to leave that up to you.

✐ JOURNAL WORK

Grab your journal and write out a list of things you not gon' do and what you will be doing instead.

CHAPTER 5

Sex and Self-Esteem

Every now and then, some self-esteem books will mention that promiscuity and poor relationships can result from or in low self-esteem. HOWEVER, they don't directly address sexuality and relationships at all! And to be perfectly honest, I am tired of it. We spend a lot of time acting like sex(uality) doesn't matter when we are talking about self-esteem, likely because so many of us have been taught that talking about sex is nasty and we see it as salacious. Kinda hard to have the whole good-girl marriageable vibe when you're talking about sex. Meanwhile, a whole bunch of us got here because someone was knocking the boots, slapping shoes, getting/giving the oochie wally, having the sex!

Baby, I'm not shy, which means that we're about to get this work going. So, in this chapter, I will speak frankly about sex and sexuality. We will talk about some of the stats, but we will also talk about how to make sure your sex life is no longer a casualty in the war against Black women's self-esteem. So, we will explore how self-esteem looks in sex, sexuality, and in romantic relationships.

Black Sex(uality) Matters!

Here is the thing: if we're talking about self-esteem, we have to also talk about sex(uality). Because if we are talking about how we feel about ourselves, and we have also been talking about how and what we know about ourselves (self-concept), then how can we not talk about sex(uality)? Especially when you consider that we are sexual beings from birth 'til death. That doesn't mean we are having sex with other people from the cradle to the grave, but it does mean we are taught and treated in a way that is gendered and sexualized from the moment someone puts a blue or pink cap on a baby's head and declares them male, female, or intersex. For some, the sexualization and gender expectations begin at the baby shower where folk have a genital, I mean gender, reveal party.

The difference between sex and sexuality is pretty easy, so we are gonna start there. Sex is what you do with your body. There are a finite number of things you can do when you are having sex because you have a finite amount of body. *Sex*, of course, also refers to what someone was assigned at birth—as in, those genitals. Do you have a vulva and vagina, or do you have a penis and scrotum? That sort of thing. *Sexuality*, on the other hand, we have already been talking about since you started reading this book. Sexuality is who you are and how you show up.[1] But here is the thing: BOTH sex and sexuality impact your self-concept and your self-esteem.

HOW DO THEY RELATE TO MY BEING BLACK?

Well, how they relate to being Black is that being a Black woman, especially a dark-skinned Black woman, we are often equated with masculinity. Furthermore, we have the tropes of the Mammy, the Jezebel, and the Sapphire to contend with. These tropes lead to the idea of an inherent sexual deviance in Black people, and especially in Black women.

Think about how dark-skinned or brown-skinned Black women are discussed. There is a way of talking about them as though they're animalistic or less than and certainly not someone to desire out loud. Back in 2016, when your girl was trying to graduate with this PhD in human sexuality, part of the work I did was in seeing how self-esteem, sexual-esteem, and hair-esteem are correlated, and baby *they were*.[2] I'm not saying they were one hundred percent correlated, but they definitely had some similarities to them. Which basically means that if your self-esteem is not rocking out, you might not be rocking out in these other spaces either.

Now, the thing about self-esteem, and sex in particular, is that regardless of where your self-esteem is, your communication in sex is impacted. When the self-concept is based on what "good girls" do, then time spent considering what you like and want becomes part of the problem. Because what we know is that for young good girls, listening to our parents without question was the norm for many of us. What followed after was listening and following directions of anyone in a place of authority, to include teachers, police, random uncles, etc. When you are a woman, this deference to authority extends to men and masculine people. As a person showing deference, having needs of your own becomes tricky shit. Tricky because your needs could then supersede someone in a space of presumed authority. Tricky because what happens when your needs differ from someone else's? If you are a "soft" and accommodating woman, then you are "supposed" to find the happy compromise—usually where you give up what you want or change what you want to fit this other person. There can be feelings of guilt associated with asking for what you want because a portion of the messaging we have received is that being a Black woman is to be undesirable. This is further exacerbated based on body size, skin tone, hair texture, facial features, and more. The idea being that the further you are from white suprem-acist beauty standards, the less desirable you are said to be. Which means a fat dark-skinned Black woman is supposed to feel lucky to be desired at all; she is not supposed to have any desire aside from pleasing her partner.

When we are unsure of ourselves, we don't communicate clearly. We try to say what we want to say while simultaneously trying to anticipate what others want to hear and considering how they will feel about what we are saying. We then adjust accordingly. As a result, we end up not saying shit. We will quite literally talk ourselves in circles, double back, change what we are saying, so that we can remain on the good foot with a partner and ease the discomfort we have been socialized to feel at being "difficult." *Difficult* in this case meaning that you are a person and are expressing needs that may oppose others of presumed authority.

On the other hand, when you are feeling yourself, when you know that you are the shit, you are more likely to show and tell others what you want. Yes, in sex, but also in life. You are more likely to advocate for yourself—especially if your self-view is not limited to a view of womanhood as defined by the male gaze for its own purpose, but rather a view of yourself as a human being with needs and desires that may differ from your lover's. You are also less likely to engage in moments of self-abandonment. *Self-abandonment*, in this case, means that you leave your wants and needs behind in order to meet the wants and needs of someone else. Which means that that whole faking it—fake moans, fake enjoyment in sex—happens a lot less. Faking it happens far more frequently when you're unsure of yourself. And being unsure of yourself is further exacerbated because so very many of us have been told that our entire worth and value is based off what somebody else wants from us, not what we want. Though, to be clear, with the way patriarchy and ideas of what a woman should be are set up, we aren't supposed to want anything from a lover other than to perform to their satisfaction.

The point is this: your sex life and your life-life are reflections of who you are, who you *think* you are, and how you feel about the combination.

✎ JOURNAL WORK

Take a moment, pause, and consider this: How's your sex life? Have you decided that faking it is easier than having another conversation about what you want or need? Have you reached a tolerable level of dissatisfaction you are willing to deal with? Or are you wanting the confidence, bravery, and words to ask for what you want? Willing to weather the storm of their feelings? To teach them your body and never fake a moan again?

A word on the "fast Black girl"

I want to add a little more into the conversation about shame, specifically as it relates to the "fast Black girl." For many of us, we were told not to wear red lipstick or red nail polish because that is the evidence of being fast. Now when it comes to the fast Black girl, as my friend Dr. Lexx Brown-James (@lexxsexdoc on Instagram) has said, "Ain't no teenage girl 'fast' enough to catch a grown man who isn't attracted to children." A whole word that, when she said it, reminded me of older men who told me that I was "mature for my age." Words that had a young me feeling myself and thinking that it meant I was ready for an "adult relationship," which was really just an inappropriate relationship with an adult. Words that further freed me and allowed space for self-forgiveness.[3]

The trope of "fast" girls gives us a sense of shame from the time that we are young because we hear things like, "Oh, you're smelling yourself," or "You think you're all that," and comments like, "Got a little bit of body, I see." The confidence or assuredness in our bodies when we are young prompts our families to place undue responsibility on us by telling us that we are fast. That we are dressing or adorning our bodies in a way that is beyond our chronological age—mind you, they bought the clothes, which means that the problem is not necessarily the clothes but rather the way the body is showing up in the clothes. The time of this supposed fastness is correlated to when the body is developing, when the little buds under your shirt start turning into actual breasts, when the thighs are a little bit thicker, when the ass is a little bit bigger. These changes, for our families, have often indicated a fastness within us. So, we learn to be ashamed of the very bodies that we have. We learn to feel like something is wrong with our bodies.

Now when we get a little bit older, the same bodies that we were told made us fast are the same bodies they expect us to use in order to catch a man. I know, very heteronormative, but that is exactly what those bodies are expected to do. We're expected to get a man so that we can get married and have babies. So, the shame around our bodies doesn't go away, but the usage of it does. Because instead of discouraging creepy uncles and nasty family friends from coming around, since they can't seem to control themselves around children, children are taught to hide themselves. Little girls are told to go get dressed because an uncle is coming. Little girls are told not to be fast. They are blamed. And so, we learn to blame ourselves in advance. The same blame carries when we are older, when we've told someone, "Stop," when

we have told someone, "No," when we have told someone, "Don't."
We are the ones blamed because we have already been seen as fast
from the time our breasts were budding. So, we carry a sense of
shame already within us, a lack of rightness that plays into how we
see ourselves. It becomes like a pair of warped glasses, distorting
the world around us and distorting the world within us.

For too many of us, our first bullies are our families, who bully
us because they know the world is unkind and that danger is
everywhere. But that doesn't make it right to place undue burden
on young shoulders, to make every woman accountable for how
men behave when we wear dresses, spaghetti straps, heels, pants,
etc. And it's not okay. But we also get to choose something different now. Because we are older. Because we are adults. Because we
don't want to pass on to our children what was given to us. But the
thing is, if we don't address that this was a problem, that we did
NOT turn out "okay," we will not change. The cycle will continue.
So, let's sit in this idea around being a fast Black girl and see if we
can unpack some of this shit. Because quiet as it's kept, some of
us say that we *were* fast Black girls. Some of us blame ourselves
for things that happened when we were growing up because we
believed that we were fast, and thus culpable.

Some of us, regardless of if fastness was bestowed upon us like
a title, will show up in the world seeing fastness in Black girls and
failing to see their humanity and curiosity, including in learning
about their bodies, learning about sex, and having a desire for
pleasure, as they take in the world around them. We judge them
from our own experiences, from what our parents gave us around

our own idea of fastness, and the ways in which America already sees sexual deviancy in the bodies of Black people, with the main condemned being Black women. So, when we see teenaged and single-digit girls dancing in cheerleading uniforms or costumes, we see them as being fast, as being too grown.

When we see Black girls with straightened hair, we say that they're being grown.

Nail polish? Grown.

Crop tops? Grown.

And that because all of these things are supposed to be so grown, these little girls must be fast and deserving of whatever will happen to them. This type of trauma is a poison to self-esteem and community care.

HOW DO SEX AND SEXUALITY RELATE TO SELF-ESTEEM?

Sex and sexuality both impact our ideas around self-concept and self-esteem. I think what we forget is that when it comes to self-concept, it's *everything* that we know about ourselves. And so much of what we think we know has already been fed to us by the propaganda machine that others have decided to place on us. When we are born, we are socialized toward someone's idea of femaleness or maleness. As a result, self-definition is already out, and we can feel a great sense of shame for the ways that we think we have failed in our performance of femaleness and/or maleness. Not to mention, since we are taught the binary, that a person should only be one or the other; people who are intersex are erased altogether—or seen as those who have failed bodily, which can create pressure to pick a side.

There are certain words that are affiliated with what it means to be a woman and to be a Black woman specifically. For women overall, there is a certain softness that we are expected to have. A willingness to be submissive, docile, quiet, adhering, a resting space, a healing place. Adding this into our tropes about strong and magical Black women, and there is an inhuman nature to consider. The part where Black women are thought of as creatures who do not need help because they can do it by themselves. Help that was never genuinely offered, because the presumed strength and independence defies the idea that you are a person who could want, let alone need, anyone's help. Besides that, there is also the idea that if you needed help, you are now a Black woman entering into the soft space of white women, the infantilized woman who requires rescuing by masculine people who protect her and provide for her, often by keeping her in the dark and deciding what she can know and what she shouldn't. This level of softness on a Black woman is often seen as a failure to live up to the strength of Black womanhood. It defies logic for some, because Blackness is so heavily associated with masculinity and imbued strength. So not only are you seen as a failure in Black womanhood, but you're also seen as someone deserving of the most bombastic side-eye that can be proffered. Black women are not seen as needing protection, so when a need for assistance, protection, or provision is seen, it reads as pathetic and manipulative.

A valuable team player

The strength and underlying masculine view doesn't release Black women to a freedom of self-determination. Nah. The womanhood part still screams: *Be of service!* The womanhood and strength come together, making Black women someone whose job and desire it should be to labor for one's family, for one's friends, to be giving and gracious to a fault. To work without question and without complaint. To give of oneself heartily and gladly. To think of oneself last, if ever. To be the strength of the family, the backbone of partners, the resting place for the weary, and the morality for all. These are things that are said to be defining characteristics for women who would be named as good and valuable. The type of women who have songs created for them. Valuable in service to others. The idea around giving and giving and giving with no end without ceasing, until one is dead.

Now, when you have this concept and idea of womanhood, of what it means to be female, how do you believe it affects our self-esteem? We're taught that we should *look* like sex but not *want* sex. That we should show up and *give* sex but never *ask for* or *receive* sex. But in the words of Summer Walker, girls need love, too! But for many of us, we are socialized to not have needs, so our self-concept is already skewed toward the ideas of what we are "supposed to" or "should" be, as opposed to who and what we actually are. When we are busy hiding portions of ourselves from view, or masking, it can be difficult to know yourself fully and integrate that self-concept.

For many of us, when we realize that pieces of ourselves are

outside of the lines of what someone else has said our femininity should look like, as a result we feel bad. We don't like those
pieces, and we are incensed when they show up in someone else,
since we have abandoned those parts of ourselves. Seeing it in
someone else feels like a slap in the face, because if we gave it up
and are living as less than we are, we expect that others should
do the same. Not to mention we worry that in being in close
proximity to another showing a piece of what we once had, we
will be exposed and called out for being just as "broken" or as
"wrong" as the person we came across. Thus begins the cycle of
policing and judging others through respectability politics. We
want to hide pieces of ourselves. We try to cloak it in certain
clothes. We try to cloak it in our righteousness and religion, in
achievement through education and academics—I mean, we are
not being called the most educated demographic for nothing,
right? We do a lot of things to try and hide pieces of ourselves
that many of us are secretly ashamed of.[4]

Yes, it relates to sex

Now, you may not think that this relates to sex, but I'm telling
you that it does. So far, we have talked about the sexuality part:
where how/what we know about ourselves comes to meet how
we feel about ourselves. When it comes sex, many of us won't
ask for what we want. We haven't even explored pleasure. We
don't touch ourselves, and we don't expect anyone else to touch
us for our pleasure or enjoyment. Some of us believe that we are

supposed to simply accept the sex that we are given and never ask for sex. And it's no wonder when Black women's sexuality has been associated with being fast, loose, or with a lack of morality. Consider being labeled "fast" for a second. What exactly was the crime? The crime was the body itself. It was the growing of breasts, the widening of hips, and the arrival of a grown woman's body on someone of our diminutive years. It made mothers, aunties, etc., tell us we were fast—a warning, an admonishment, and an attempt to keep us safe. It inspired those same folk to tell us to cover our bodies when uncles were coming over. It inspired grown folk to place adult gazes at the center and shame us accordingly. We were shamed simply for having bodies that had the audacity to grow. How, then, does it look when we ask for something? If we say we want sex and how we want the sex, how we want to feel during sex, we haven't properly performed femininity and we have now shown ourselves to be what our mamas once called us. Some of us have yet to explore any of these concepts, because our self-esteem is hanging in the balance. If we say what we want, if we go after it joyfully, then we're whores, with the hard R. And if we're whores, how do we feel about ourselves, especially when others have already told us there is no value in an unvirtuous woman?

Some of us want to dress and adorn our bodies, much like Cardi B on a stage would. We want the BBLs. We want the breast implants. We want the liposuction, the Coke bottle body and to adorn that body in all kinds of fashions. And yet, we also understand that people judge us according to what we wear, stripping us down to a one-dimensional character who could only be for sex. We worry about the judgment. And for many of us, we adjust accordingly. That is part of sex and sexuality. How people sexualize our bodies based on what we wear, how we look in what we wear, and the assumptions about our character that stem from it. As though only goodness can flow if you wear a suit and only salaciousness follows from bodysuits and red heels.

I don't know if you remember newscaster bae Demetria Obilor from back in 2017. She was a morning traffic reporter at a local news station WFAA in Dallas, Texas, who went viral. She was wearing a dress that went from collarbone to knee but because she got bawdy-ody, she was judged and called names, told that she was provocative and salacious. Women's bodies are already sexualized. Black women's bodies, more so. If you have a bigger butt, if you have bigger breasts, ain't no hiding that in your clothes. So many of us try to hide pieces of our sexuality. We try to hide the very bodies that we have, because we have learned to be ashamed of them from our parents to church to society at large.

If you think this does not impact how you show up in sex, or when it is time to have sex, you are sadly mistaken. Some of us will only have sex in the dark because we're afraid that what we are doing should not be seen in the light, that our bodies should not be seen by our partners and enjoyed. We are ashamed to see our own bodies. Some of us have learned to care for our bodies in the most basic ways possible, specifically keeping it clean. Because we learn that cleanliness is next to godliness, we wash our bodies, but we don't enjoy them. We don't touch them. We don't celebrate them. We don't revere them. We don't worship at the altar of our bodies. We don't revel in the way that our bodies experience pleasure, and I do mean all kinds of sensuous pleasure, not just sexual pleasure. Sex and pleasure can go hand in hand, but it requires a purposefulness that we don't display. We ignore and distrust our bodies so heavily that we won't eat when we're hungry. We won't consider what foods taste delicious on our tongues and make us want to dance (or is it just me?), and so we move similarly when it comes to sex. We are disconnected and disgusted. We believe that sex is something that we give to a partner. And maybe in return they will give us orgasms, a relationship, and kids, giving away any sense of responsibility for our desires. Placing others in charge as though our orgasms are not our responsibility. As though our pleasure is not our responsibility. And as though our pleasure is really made for partners and not for us. But a capitalistic society has already convinced us that ALL bodies are made for labor. That Black and brown bodies should labor for whiteness. That women's bodies should additionally labor for men. We are at an intersectional laboring and usage of bodies in ways that do not honor us and thus cannot be made for pleasure.

This is why I started Plan to Orgasm—it's a masterclass, yes, but also a retreat. The whole point is that we want to have pleasure in the bedroom, but we also want to have pleasure in life. Some of us just don't know that we're deserving of this pleasure because we don't *feel* deserving. Because our self-concept, and the idea of "who we are for," has been warped. If you're only for other people, if you're only in service to your parents, if you're only in service to your partner, then you're never in service to you. This means that your pleasure and how you feel about sex doesn't matter. And for me, a whole sex therapist, it is a sadness to believe that our lives are only meant for others.

☕ TEA TIME

Now, here's the thing, I'm not exempt. It has been pounded into me that as a Nigerian woman, my job was to keep house, cook, and care for kids. Despite my not believing that. My actions were incongruent with my thoughts. My partner and I moved in together, and I moved into a role of service to make his life easier. It took reflection and time to let go of what I had been taught and get back into my seat of pleasure. I didn't need to be in service to my partner in that way. It made me miserable. I was stressed out. It's hard to be authentically you when the you you are performing is a service bot divorced from her body and desires. The transition from the desires of others to my desires was uncomfortable, painful, and scary. It was filled with anxiety, depression, and a lack of assuredness. But I followed my body, trusted my gut and my ability to reason, asked for what I needed, and spoke my desires. I am well on my way even if I am not there yet. It is a lifelong journey, not something you achieve on a Tuesday and never have to work at again.

Supremacy culture is pervasive and ever evolving. At the moment, supremacy culture is about maintaining power and control of women, Black folk, and people of color through requiring us to be chaste, clean, and of service. It's about earning value through productivity and self-control, through denying a need or desire for rest or pleasure. So, we don't rest. We don't take what we need, and we don't revel in pleasure except on the weekends—when we feel that we have earned it. This especially relates to being Black. As Black women, specifically, we use our bodies and lives as the evidence to display our adherence to the politics of respectability. When you add this into the ideas around sexual promiscuity that are often attributed to Black bodies—the Jezebel, the Sapphire, the Mammy, and the Black Buck (for men/masculine folk), we can feel like there is much to prove. That our bodies are meant to be in service, an ongoing apology for existing in melanin and estrogen, which means we are never meant to be in pleasure. This impacts how we feel about ourselves. Some of us don't feel good about ourselves because we don't experience any sort of pleasure. And when we do feel pleasure, we feel guilty about it. Our self-esteem suffers. We move into a space of low self-esteem because we're trying to use our bodies to prove our worth to someone else whom we want to give us praise so that we can feel good about ourselves.

When your pleasure, when your happiness, when all of these things are in someone else's pocket, they're not yours to command. When they're in someone else's pocket, that person has control of whether or not you get to feel good about yourself and about whether or not you get to experience pleasure. I think, quite honestly, it's the one thing that I have enjoyed about the pandemic:

the part where everyone was home, and every sex toy was sold. Where there was more exploration of one's body, where people were taking their pleasure and talking about it just a little bit more openly. As we have moved back to business as normal, a lot of us have moved away from rest. We've moved back into burnout, and we've moved away from pleasure. We're back into the idea that pleasure is that thing that you earn after you've worked hard Monday through Friday. So, Friday night, Saturday, and a portion of your Sunday get to be in a space of pleasure. And then your Sunday afternoon and evening are dedicated to getting ready for Monday. This is a sadness. But I can see the role of capitalistic, patriarchal, and white supremacist *shoulds*.

How should you show up as a woman? How should you show up as a Black woman? And how does your sex play a role in that? How should you cover your body? How should your body be adorned? How should you seek pleasure with your body, or should you seek it at all? How should you show up for your partner sexually? Because part of it is "what you don't do, another woman will." All of these things show up in our sex lives and all of these things impact how we know ourselves and how we feel about ourselves—whether or not we are deserving of pleasure and how we get to interact with others. However, like rest, pleasure is not earned. It is simply taken when you desire it. And as Sonya Renee Taylor has said, the body is not an apology.

◌ JOURNAL WORK

So, here's a little homework for you. I know that we can't begin truly communicating with others about sex until we also start communicating with ourselves around sex. So here is a QR code.

Go grab my yes/no/maybe list. Now, this list contains several sexual acts that you can either try solo or with a partner. Some of them obviously require a partner, but a lot of them can be done solo, and I just want you to take a moment to consider what you like, what you don't like, and what you've never done. Consider how you might explore yourself. And I understand that a lot of us also have shame around sex. That's why I created the *30 Day Masturbation Guide* and a corresponding class. I realize that shame around sex can be debilitating.

But here's the good news. Did you know that masturbation as well as having sex that you want to have can increase your feelings of self-esteem? It helps you feel better about you. Partly because you're learning more about your body, how your body responds to pleasure, and how you lean into trusting the feeling and letting go. And all of these as far as I'm concerned are life lessons. Learning to listen to your inner voice, to be in alignment with your body, to know when your body wants rest, when it wants food, when it wants water, when it needs sex. This is a part of knowing yourself; this is self-concept. Then, giving yourself what you need and feeling good about it helps to increase our sense of self-esteem. I don't want us to keep losing in that area.

Consent and Sex Acts

I am not gonna say too much here, because this has been partially covered in Chapter 4. Here is the thing, when it comes to consent, things look very different on a Black woman's body than they do on anyone else's. Everyone believes it is their right to have access to Black bodies, from people wanting to reach out and touch our hair in the streets, to people thinking they should have access to our bodies between the sheets. Ownership of our bodies is a daily battle as the world around us regulates women's fertility, and as some men lament their lack of access to the women they desire because they have failed to be desirable to us.

Keeping up with what was already presented in the fast Black girl section, consider this: If you start off life with people believing that you are fast, do you think it changes when you are older? The answer is no. Everyone thinks they should have power and control over someone else. White folk think they should have dominion over all people of color and Black folk. Men believe they should have dominion over women and feminine folk. Parents think they should have dominion over their kids. People with money think they should have dominion over folk who do not. I could keep going, but I will stop here. The point is that people in positions of power believe that their power should be flexed, not on themselves, but on people who are different from themselves.

Sexually, this shows up in how people steal another person's choice through sexual assault. Touching someone without their permission, raping someone. We have often heard people talk about rape as though it is about pleasure. That the person is simply seeking pleasure. But this is NOT true. Rape is about the expression of power and feeling powerful. It's about subverting the will of someone else to put your own in its place. And Black women are thought of as fast, sexually deviant, and undesirable. The Jezebel can't be raped because her sexual expression (in just being) is seen as masculine in its hypersexuality. For her, you are doing a favor. The Mammy, with her dark skin and vastness of body, she is so undesirable that you are doing her a favor. And for the Sapphire, with her attitude, you are reminding her of her place—working to make her submissive. All excuses to place innocence where it does not exist.

These tropes play out in the public sphere in the "What was she wearing?" and "Why was she there?" narratives seeking to find explanation for actions for which there will never be an excuse, or to determine that the crime was the body being denied to someone else.

The point: Black women have not had the same access to consent as white counterparts. And because of the nature of white supremacy, we are less likely to report it because Black men are already unfairly targeted, white folk rarely convict one of their own, and there is a lack of belief in Black women because we were once "fast Black girls" who had the audacity to grow into sexually deviant (e.g., sexually curious, wanting, and healthy) adults.

This burden doesn't belong to us, nor should we keep it. I know Issa Rae said she is for everybody Black, but anyone who wants to play in our faces can fuck around and find out. Your *no* is not something that needs to be stated and restated for someone to hear it. Your being "not interested" is not an invitation to try harder or disregard your will. They need to hear you. You deserve pleasure and safety, especially in the body that you occupy.[5]

Courting, Dating, and Long-Term Relationships

SHAME SHAME SHAME AND PICKING PARTNERS

I've said it before, and I'll say it again: shame spawns secrets. When we feel ashamed of ourselves, we are not feeling guilty. Guilt is productive. Guilt tells us that we did something wrong. But shame tells us that something is wrong with *us*. And when it comes to sex and sexuality, many of us feel ashamed. We feel ashamed of our desires. We feel ashamed of the things that we want to do. We feel ashamed of the things that we have done. We feel ashamed of the people we have been with and how many. And when it comes to that, what happens is that it then spawns a certain level of secrecy. We will not only tell *others* lies, but we tell *ourselves* lies, too. We tell ourselves why we did or didn't do whatever we did. We lie and tell ourselves that someone we had sex with was the best sex of our lives and that's why we keep returning to them, instead of saying we are scared to add to our "body count." We are spinning an epic tale of how we will be single if we don't go back to an ex who we already know is not a good fit for us. We try to hide because we don't want to be judged by others because we're worried about how they will look at us. So, we lie.

Now, the thing is, when we lie, we tell ourselves a completely different story about the person we are. Which means that some of us see ourselves as broken, nasty, disgusting people. We see ourselves as people not worthy of what we desire. Because the shame and the secrets have spawned lies that we tell ourselves and that we kinda tell others. Some of us will enter the fake-it-'til-we-make-it stage, where we will pretend that everything is all good. But the thing is, the lies that we believe about ourselves are still going to come out in our actions. And some of us will pretend, some of us will just be in the space where we are just upset in ourselves, and we will allow shame to make our decisions. For some of us, that means that we pick our partners according to our secret shame. We pick partners who we think will accept our shame, but never tell them about it. We pick partners who revile our shame so that we can keep ourselves in line. The point is, though, that shame helps us to pick our partners, helps us to pick our behaviors, consciously and unconsciously. Ultimately, it doesn't serve us in our sexuality or in our sex because when we're feeling shame, we don't ask for what we want; instead, we take what we are given. Sometimes, we may even remind our partners that certain sexual acts are nasty, even when we are curious to try them. Sometimes we allow shame to be the thing that chooses for us whether or not we're going to be celibate or chaste until marriage or some other predetermined time, and then decide what type of sexual acts we are allowed to partake in. Despite the fact that even the church says the marriage bed is undefiled. The point is that shame is pervasive and impacts what we see about ourselves and how we feel about what we see.

THERE IS, INDEED, PISS IN THE DATING POOL

I have heard time and again that there is piss in the dating pool. If someone told you that there are plenty of fish in the sea, you would also remind them that there is also plenty of trash, too. Baby, you ain't wrong, per se, but you might be without all the information.

Here is the thing, everyone is in various stages of personal development. Some actually seek it out and some wait for life to beat them upside the head and force a change. And yes, there are those who will never do anything different than what they have been doing. But let me say this: we have to be honest with ourselves; some of us are also choosing to be with people we know from the jump are not a good fit. I know, it sounds like I am blaming the fisherman for pulling up garbage in the net, but that's because you haven't heard me well. I am not blaming you for attracting everyone to you. I am saying that you have to take responsibility for keeping the shit that doesn't fit you.

You are not a magnet for fuckfolk. You are a magnet that attracts everyone. They all wanna be in your presence, whether or not you know what it is that you are bringing into the space. Whether or not you know how it is that you are shining. Whether or not you know you're the shit. Some want to just bask in the glory of you; some want to possess you; others want to see what makes you shine and if you would be willing to dim your light so they can say they have had you. All people have an agenda when they tryna be or get close to you. The problem is not what they want; the problem is what you keep. When you see red flag after red flag, do you toss that fish back into the sea or do you keep it and try to make a fricassée of it? When you have set a boundary and see that the person you're with won't even pretend like they respect it, do you say, "Cool beans, you do you; imma do me...over there"? Or do you try to make it work and find the compromise to your boundaries? Do you collect fuckbois and fuckgirls like Ash Ketchum collected Pokémon?

There are over seven billion people on the planet. Over five hundred million people in North America. Did I mention that over two hundred million of those people are over twenty-one? Please go play in someone else's face and tell them that there is only trash. Because if there is only trash out there, then you must be counting yourself among the garbage. Why? Cuz people are tryna date you, too!

Part 2

MIND YOUR MATTER

At this point, we move into section two of the book. There is a quote that says something like fifty percent of success is inspiration, and the other fifty percent is perspiration. I would hope that by this point, we should be at around fifty percent inspiration. We have intimate knowledge, and that can inspire us to do some work. So, now we move!

So far, we have gotten really deep into understanding what makes up self-esteem and all the ways we are impacted by it. What

I like about Part 1 of this book most of all is that, while I have asked you to take responsibility for your healing, I have already noted that we don't get hurt in isolation. But what I like about Part 2 is that we move from the part where we *know* better, to where we *do* better. If you think knowing better was a doozy, then be fore-warned that doing better is a whole other ballgame.

So, how do we get to doing the actual work? Well, I suggest remembering one thing: this is going to be difficult. It is going to feel "not right," but that's only because it's unfamiliar. To assist us, we make sure we have accountability partners and friends who we can talk to. I also suggest having a list of coping skills to lean on when you are feeling like it's all too much. If you find it necessary, get a therapist on board.

A few other things to remember: While we are doing the work, we are not comparing ourselves to where we think others are or where we "should" be. This is not a competition. The folk around you are in collaboration for healing. It's not that you are trying to "get to" the destination of healing before anyone else. So, this is where I bring my momma back into it and remind you, as she reminded me, to "face your front." Take your time, read this part through, go back armed with a highlighter, and when you work it, do so with community.

Please remember that "healed" is not a destination. Healing is not linear, and it is very likely never done. This process is cyclical, nonlinear, and hard AF. Besides that, moving in new ways is a habit that has to be built over time. The same way you were in thoughtless patterns of self-hurt, it takes time to build up patterns of self-healing. If it took you thirty years to get here, to a place where you are ready to heal, then please don't get down on yourself for not "figuring it out" and "getting it right" in a few days. That's not even fair. Remember, healing is a process, but it does require you to mind your matter. You got this!

.

CHAPTER 6

Becoming the Bob the Builder of Boundaries

I had this client, let's call her Brittany, and she was beautiful. Dark skin, kinky hair with blond tips, thicker than a Snickers, funny, and anxious as hell. By that, I mean the anxiety was intense enough that going to work made her want to throw up. She would talk about the pressure she was feeling but that no one else seemed to see. And why couldn't they see it? Because Brittany was excellent—in every sense of the word. She was a supervisor at her job, a great friend, an attentive daughter, and a protective sister to her siblings. No one could see how anxious she was or how much she was doubting herself. The thing is, Brittany had very permissive loosey-goosey boundaries. If you needed something, she was on it. Even if no one asked for anything, she was always proactive, considerate of others' issues, and ready to meet their needs.

As a result, her anxiety grew. She was falling asleep on her couch because she stayed up too late. Dragging herself to bed at two or three in the morning, hitting the snooze button three times too many the next morning. Rushing through her routine to be on time for work. Only to feel the anxiety rising the closer she got to the building. It was a repetitive loop and getting old.

She said to me: "I can't live like this."

She meant it, which meant we had to work on her boundaries.

We've spent a lot of time in the previous chapters talking about the components that make up self-esteem and how the world around us impacts it. After all that discussion, I still have to ask: Do you think we can build a life we enjoy and delight in without boundaries? The answer is that you can't. It's hard to build a life based on *you* without boundaries.

Without boundaries, we're destined to find ourselves stuck in a loop. In this loop, all we want is for other people to see us as useful and good—that way, we can see ourselves (at least temporarily) as likable—but we lack self-knowledge. Staying in this loop can leave us feeling anxious, depressed, angry, resentful, and ultimately *tired*. In this chapter, we'll talk about what boundaries are, how to stop the mentality that says, *Fuck it, I'll do it*, and how boundaries impact how we are able to build and maintain our healthy self-concept and self-esteem, and I'll give you some more in-depth boundary-building resources! This first chapter in the Mind Your Matter section is moving into more doing. Please don't get so caught up in the reading that you forget you have to DO this book.

What Are Boundaries?

When it comes to healing self-esteem, one of the things that we often need to practice is setting and maintaining boundaries. Baby, many of us have porous boundaries—boundaries that are based on the comfort and happiness of everyone *except* for us. We've spent our time, we've used our energy, we've allowed people to use our bodies, we've made space for the emotional dumper, we've allowed parents to place undue burden on us (perceiving their expectations as primary whether they're financial, physical, etc.), and so much more.

According to the *Merriam-Webster Dictionary*, a boundary is "something that indicates or fixes a limit or extent."

As for me and my house, I define boundaries as the lines that differentiate you and what's for you from someone else and what's for them. Knowing that difference between what's for *you* and what's for *them* contributes to the mental, emotional, and physical wellness that allows you to have relationships in a way that keeps you feeling healthy, safe, and sane. It's the space between how you govern yourself and how someone else governs themselves. Things get murky when you try to govern someone else (or they are trying to govern you) without either of you remembering that you're different people with different needs.

If you think of boundaries as a property line between houses, as Dr. Henry Cloud and Dr. John Townsend say in *Boundaries in Marriage*, then boundaries are the space where you can do what you want—so long as you don't adversely impact or interfere with your neighbor, and vice versa.[1] It helps you to know who is responsible for what.

Like in *Super Mario Bros.*, there are levels to this shit. What I mean is that boundaries occur in all kinds of relationships. You have boundaries for yourself as an individual; your family has boundaries against those who are not of blood relation; your family may also have further boundaries within itself (for you and your siblings, for you and your parents); your teams at work may have them; your friends probably have them, too. Boundaries are everywhere!

With boundaries, I would be remiss if I didn't name the various kinds of boundaries you can think about. I won't say this is exhaustive, but there are six categories of boundaries to consider:

1. **Physical Boundaries:** relating to personal space, touch, and other things for your body (like food, rest, water, using the bathroom, etc.)

2. **Intellectual Boundaries:** relating to your mind (your thoughts, imaginings, ideas, etc.)

3. **Time Boundaries:** how much time you give in various settings (whether it be at work, in conversation with a friend, or anywhere else)

4. **Material Boundaries:** relating to your stuff (anything physical like a car, house, favorite sweater, or book) and respecting those things, choosing how, when, and if you share them

5. **Emotional Boundaries:** relating to how we allow others to treat us (without calling in disrespect), and to respect for and honoring emotions and emotional energy

6. **Sexual Boundaries:** relating to consent and respect of preferences, desires, and privacy

Within these areas, your boundaries can be **POROUS** (like cheese paper—people go right through them). They can be **RIGID** (like the Great Wall of China—so high, wide, and long that there is no give to them). Or they can be **HEALTHY-ISH** (like the fence of a house—the boundary is clearly marked, and only certain folks have the ability come on to the property).

Personal boundaries are just that, *personal.* Your boundaries are going to look different from other people's boundaries. But often we find ourselves judging people's boundaries, saying what *we* believe is reasonable or unreasonable, usually based on how convenient those boundaries are with respect to what *we* want. But that math is not mathing! Boundaries are developed in private and practiced in public. Every interaction you have is a way to learn what feels good and what doesn't. In your alone time, when you reflect on the day you had and about what was working (or what was working your nerves), you may be better able to see what kind of boundary you need, when you need them, and with whom you need to enforce them. Healthy boundaries are based on what you know about you and your needs. Healthy boundaries are taught through what someone does and says and how they behave.

INSPIRED PEOPLE

Remember this: we are largely self-centered people. We often think that others do (or should) think like we do and see things the way we do. We take on the leading role in our lives—we are the sun of our personal universe—and as a result, we can think the world revolves around us, that the other characters' lives are merely about moving our story along. This is still true when it comes to boundaries and how we enact or don't enact them. When we lack healthy boundaries, we're inspired to believe others should also not have boundaries. On the other hand, when we have rigid AF boundaries, we also believe that this is true or should be true for other people.

The world around us is rife with examples of a lack of boundaries—of holding them or respecting them. Jobs often lack time-based boundaries, requiring you to show that you are a team player by giving more time than is due to them. They judge you based on how much extra you're willing to give at no additional cost to them. So, these jobs will reward or punish you based on time that doesn't belong to them. Jobs benefit from folk without boundaries. Those people are upheld as examples of having a good work ethic, and it inspires supervisors to believe all folk who work there should behave similarly.

☕ *TEA TIME*

Let me grab a tea bag real quick... I was working for an agency (to remain unnamed) back in the day in the DMV area. Apparently, word was getting around from my supervisor to all that I was "difficult to work with." Their thought was, since I had no children and no husband, that I had no barriers preventing me from working late or coming in early as requested. I was pretty strict about my time. I wanted to work my forty hours, no more—and less if I could have it. Well, my supervisor went on leave, and I was temporarily reassigned to someone else, who I should say, was worried about working with me, because everyone thought I was difficult. In my time with her, when she asked me to do something late/after hours, I said yes, but that I would need the time back. She thought that was perfectly reasonable—that was when she let it slip about my being difficult. She said something like, "You're a lot easier to work with than I expected." And there were the beans, spilled all over the floor. They had unreasonable expectations of my time, that I should never request overtime payment or get my time back, because it was expected of me to be a "team player" by giving up time as requested. They didn't know I was in school earning my PhD (it wasn't their business). They didn't know I was dating a geographically undesirable person (it also wasn't their business). They didn't know about my home life because, say it with me, IT. WASN'T. THEIR. BUSINESS! But because some organizations believe you to be their property, they also think that every hour of every day should be dedicated to them. That you should prove your loyalty by over-giving your time, your energy, or whatever the hell else they want. So, they will require you to violate your boundaries and call it "being a team player," even though they would gladly fire you on a Friday *after* you've worked all day or right before a holiday. Quiet as it's kept, some of us treat friends, lovers, and others like the job treats us. But I digress.

THE JOY IN HEARING NO

There can be joy in hearing other people say *no* and protect their peace. I know, it sounds WILD, but it's true. Too many of us say yes when we don't want to, and we end up quietly resenting people who ask us for things. When someone is sitting in their boundaries and enforcing them, you will find that this person says *no—not yet, maybe later, never, etc.*—a whole lot more. The best part about it is that on some level, it means that they know themselves *and* that they are sharing themselves with you. They trust themselves to hold their peace, but they also trust you to have enough respect for them to not cross the line they have drawn. That's love.

I asked a friend of mine to read something I was writing—no, not for this book. They told me no. I was a little hurt, because I wanted their opinion, but I also respected their no. They didn't have the mental or emotional space to give. While I wanted their opinion, and it is important to me, I also value their well-being more than I value how they can be of service to me. The best part is this: when I asked for something else later and they said yes, I knew they meant it. I didn't have to question if they were giving me pity or if they were neglecting something on their end. I knew they had the time and wanted to spend it with me because they had a history of expressing and holding their boundaries to protect their mental and emotional health. What I am saying is that boundaries can ultimately foster trust. Trust that the person who tells you no is taking care of themselves, and trust in you as a person who respects their boundaries. It gives us all a little more room to show up authentically.

How Are Boundaries Important to Self-Esteem?

So, my girl Brittany, with all her do-for-others shit, was always tired and anxious. But when she started implementing boundaries, she had the space to know more about herself. She learned when she had more energy and when she didn't. She realized which friendships felt good, genuine, and like they had reciprocity, and when ones felt draining, discouraging, and like a one-way street of her being the giver. This allowed her more space to consider what she wanted her mental and emotional climate to be during the day and behave accordingly. It meant that she didn't speak to certain people before work, so she felt less stressed. It meant that she implemented a quiet hour when she got to work so she could organize her day and tackle priorities quicker. It meant creating a routine that involved decompressing, being with friends, and having a nighttime routine, instead of helping people and then watching Netflix in a stupor on her couch. The more she learned about herself, the more she was able to see that she needed boundaries to order her life and protect her peace.

The best part for me, as her therapist, was seeing the impact it had on her self-esteem. She started paying closer attention to how she felt watching certain shows and movies—removing things that made her feel bad about her chocolate skin and her body shape—including culling the social media accounts she was following. She had tough conversations with friends about feeling used, telling them what she felt was off in their relationship and how they could get back on track, from her perspective, and asking them for theirs. I remember her coming to therapy saying, "I am feeling good in my body." She noticed she was sleeping better, she was engaged when she was with people, and she was feeling better overall. She still didn't like her job, but she stopped having panic attacks in the parking lot. She still had some work to do, but she stopped feeling overwhelmed by everything all the time.

Boundaries are not just a way for you to say *no* or *fuck you* to the people in your life. They are a way for you to acknowledge the space between where others end and where you begin. Boundaries are a way to determine what feels good and safe to enter your space, and to remove the things that don't—or at least limit your contact or employ some strategies around them.

✐ JOURNAL WORK

Write a list of twenty things you know about yourself. This can help bring you back to the fact that you do know yourself and help you when it comes to building those boundaries.

Self-concept: what we know about ourselves very much impacts how we feel about ourselves. Too many of us don't really know ourselves because we are always and constantly in service of others. Boundaries give you more space to learn about you and consider how you are with others. Now, I know the extrovert is likely thinking, *But that's where I get my energy!* And they're right—it is! There's no denying that. AND there are strategies that the extrovert can learn from the introvert and vice versa. One of those strategies being to chill out and consider how you feel with each interaction and what you might want to change on your end and ask for from the person on the other end.

🍵 TEA TIME

My boundaries were absolute TRASH in the height of the panini. I had really good boundaries before it, but then really poor ones in it. I was a solo practitioner at the time, and I wanted to help everyone who was coming to me for therapy. I said yes to every opportunity to speak online—even if I didn't much like the topic or the audience wasn't quite the right fit for me. I was saying yes to more clients, saying yes to more family time, and saying yes to trying things I wasn't particularly interested in. Add my shenanigans to the fear and anxiety I had about contracting COVID, and it pushed me to being a real heaping mess of nerves. I had a hard time concentrating, I felt on edge much of the time, and I was always fucking tired. This made me more sensitive to loud noises—and that Fourth of July was brutal because I swear the fireworks must have been ten for one dollar the way they were lighting them up for weeks before and after the Fourth. Captain Doing Too Much needed a break!

Implementing boundaries, doing my self-reflection work at the end of the day (or the week), talking to my therapist, and creating routines for waking up and going to bed all helped me to better see the ways I was ignoring myself. It helped me to see what my needs were and what I needed to do to get back to and stay in my homeostasis. Learning what I needed and implementing it, saying *no* or *not yet* to the folk asking me for things, referring people to other therapists, and then hiring a therapist to join my team helped me immensely. Delegating tasks and learning how to ask my partner, family, and friends for help were some of the key things to my success in dealing with my anxiety and creating boundaries. Now I can tell you, I ain't doing shit by myself that I ain't got to do by myself, and I check in on my boundaries and communicate as necessary. It helps me to like myself better and to like the folk I fuck with, too.

STOPPING THE "FUCK IT, I'LL DO IT," MENTALITY

Something that seems to happen just a bit too often is the "Fuck it, I'll do it" mentality. This was something Brittany also was on. If something needed to be done for the family, she tried to get volunteers or coordinate; if folk were moving too slow or not doing it how she wanted it done, she would throw up her hands and say, "Fuck it, I'll do it." She said it guaranteed that the work would be done to her standards. Though she was not the mule of the world, she was def feeling like the mule of her family. Her value was derived from her labor and how she gave to others—a concept that for many people can also offer a sense of pride and self-worth relative to others. And boy was she feeling that. She felt a sense of pride in both her ability to get things done and the way she was known in her family as the one who gets things done.

Even if this is not exactly your story, it doesn't mean you are not out here participating as the quarterback for Team Doing Too Much!

To be the backbone, glue, or doer of the family can feel like constantly having to do things because others will not be able to do it right because of their actual incompetence or their weaponized incompetence. *Weaponized incompetence* is when someone intentionally does something poorly in order to get someone else to do it, thereby getting themselves off the hook, teaching you not to ask them in the future and adding more work to your plate.[2] People in your life may often say things like "You got it" or "You got this" as a way to note that even if you're asking for help, you don't really need it.

We have been indoctrinated into this hyperindividualism, which is actually a show of one's trauma. So, we say, "Fuck it, I'll do it." And do it, we do. We will kinda ask for help, but give no indication of what we need or how someone can be an asset to us.

This traps us into constantly being in motion *doing something* in a hyperindividualistic mindset and bars us from being in community with others. Learning to trust others to get something done is the goal, even if they don't do it exactly the way that you would have. The goal is being able to see and appreciate the variety in how people think and how they accomplish tasks.

Here's the thing: this is an *us* problem, not necessarily a *them* problem. We have dubbed ourselves the "strong friend." The doer of the group. Captain Save a Hoe. Be honest, it can feel nice to be needed. It can make us feel important, and it feels demonstrative of our strength. The problem we have is the same one that Superman has. The same one that Metro Man had in the movie *Megamind*—when you make it your job to swoop in and save the day, you also disempower the people around you to save themselves. Let that soak in. We are so helpful and doing such a great job that others around us can be stunted in the face of all our greatness. We don't make it easy for the people around us to even develop the executive skills we have, then we blame them for its lack of development taking the tasks for ourselves while we are throwing up our hands saying, "Fuck it."

Being the helpful one, the one with your shit together, can also be a whole-assed identity and a way to hide shame. If we feel like something is wrong with us, that we are secretly damaged, we may try to cover up those insecurities by trying to do more. But remember what I said back in Chapter 3? You cannot DO your way into liking yourself.

Let this be a reflection moment: Are you wearing your Captain Save a Hoe cape? Because Edna Mode already said NO CAPES!

✐ JOURNAL WORK

STRATEGY TO IMPLEMENT: PRACTICE ASKING.

Ask one person to help you with or do something for you today (or tomorrow, depending on what time it is). It can be something small, large, or in between. Tell them what you need, when you need it, and then sit your ass down. Allow them to do it. If they don't get it done, that's on them, not you. If they do, they are showing you they can rise to the challenge...if you let them.

Identifying the Boundaries You Need to Set and with Whom

Some say that identifying the boundaries you need is the most difficult or even the most important part of the boundary-having process. Clearly, I disagree, since I did not put this section first. The most important part to me is knowing you need the boundaries in the first place. The second part is knowing *why* you need those boundaries. Knowing your why makes it more likely that you will follow through or even that you will return to them when you abandon those boundaries for whatever reason.

Brittany, when she was ready to set boundaries, couldn't, for the life of her, figure out where she needed to actually set them. Not to mention she simply thought boundaries meant telling everyone no all the time. Most of us have a view of boundaries as something negative because boundaries are seen as negative in our culture. There is an encouraged culture of permissiveness that really is only detrimental to the people who are not in power. The folk in positions of power also have boundaries that naturally come with their position baked into the structures that make them so-called "more powerful" than us.

Off the top of my head, here are some of the relationships and spaces where you might need to set a few boundaries. These are the ones Brittany needed, and I've told you some of my tea, so some of this is also what I needed. Since my family might read this book, I won't tell you which are from my experience or which are from Brittany's experience. I am also gonna throw some extras in there from other clients, friends, and from my imagination for a little razzle-dazzle.

In the first few items of this list, you will find people. Those are people you may need to set a boundary with. Other parts of the list relate to situations, personal information, and your things (time included).

→ Momma

→ Friends

→ Papa

→ Uncles

→ Aunties

→ Siblings

→ Your significant (or not so significant) other

→ Your dwelling (house, apartment, whatever)

→ Your vehicle

→ Response to texts and emails

→ Time of day you will engage

→ Mealtimes

→ Comments about your appearance

→ Your marital status

→ Your child creation desires and status

→ Borrowing things from you

→ Staying in your place

→ Your time

→ Your assistance with stuff (like airport drop-offs and pick-ups)

→ How someone can treat you

→ How someone can speak to you

→ Holiday gatherings

→ Family vacations

→ Work

→ Sex you're willing to have, when, and with whom

→ The boundary line of your home property

This list is not exhaustive, but it can be a great starting place.

✐ JOURNAL WORK

Try placing a star next to the ones you think you may need to reevaluate boundaries for. After you know where boundaries are needed, pick the one item from the list that has been the most bothersome for you recently. Consider what is bothering you about your interaction in that space. Take a moment to feel it out. How do you often feel in that space or with those people? And why do you feel that way? Then consider: What would *you* need to do to feel better? Consider if these are people you can talk to about what you need in order to feel safer and saner. If they are folk you can talk to, what are the three major points you want to bring up in that discussion? When will you ask them to have that discussion, making sure that you both (or all) block off enough time to move through it? What actions can you take for yourself that can help you maintain your emotional and mental wellness? (Remember, I am asking what you *can* do because your boundaries are your responsibility. It marks what you need to do, not what rule you want to place on someone else.)

Another way you can figure out your needs and begin setting boundaries is to start with your values and desires. What do you value in your life? What do you want to have more of or less of? With Brittany, she wanted to feel like she knew what she wanted in romantic relationships. She had a desire to get married, have a couple of kids, and move back to her hometown so she could not only give but receive more support from her family.

Once she understood that her values are family, support, sharing, peace, ease, sleep, friends, and physical comforts, she was able to see the ways she was and was not living in accordance with those values. She was able to see, for example, that the "nice enough" guy she was dating didn't really fit in—and that he wasn't all that nice. She was also able to see that while her job afforded her physical comforts because it paid well, it didn't offer her a sense of peace, ease, or support. Now, don't get it twisted; she didn't just up and quit, but she did make a plan to transition over the next year and a half from that job to a part-time job that largely consisted of work she liked to do and starting up her own business, which would offer her more time and freedom to engage in the other aspects she desired.

Her values guided her on the path to healthier boundaries, supported by her self-knowledge, which helped with the healing and growth of her self-esteem. An all-around win!

Communicating Boundaries with Others

"But I don't know what to say."

I get it. When it comes to telling others about our boundaries, we may struggle to find the right words. But here's the thing: you *do* know what to say; you're just worried about hurting someone's feelings or how they are going to take it. And I get that. However, sometimes those boundaries need to be communicated with our inner asshole. Now, I am not saying go *be* an asshole; I am saying that we will talk ourselves into circles so ridiculous that no one will know what you are trying to say at all.

So, when it comes to telling someone about your boundaries follow these tips:

1. Use short declarative sentences.
2. Bring it back to elementary. Tell them what you need to say, give supporting statements if you want to, and restate what you said at the start.
3. Write it down or practice if you're feeling nervous.

☕ TEA TIME

Here is some tea time to get you started. I love my momma. I think she is the bee's knees. She is funny, smart, chill, and also a member of a Team Doing Too Much since 1963. My momma is supportive and nosey. Delightful and pushy. Chill and a whole-assed busybody. When it came to my wedding, my momma was over the top. I know she wanted it to be done well and she wanted to help, but I felt like I was going nuts. So, I asked for support from my sisters, told my mom what I needed, and made sure to consider what I required for me so I could maintain my peace. I created schedule times when I was open to talking about the wedding and when I was not. I would start off conversations with my momma by stating if it was wedding convo time or naw, and I asked that she respect it. When she strayed, I warned her. But if she just needed to do it and I wasn't in the space for it, I would tell her I had to go and would call her later. My sisters were asked to be filters, according to their boundaries. If momma was talking about doing or buying something, she needed to tell them first, and they would let her know if it was something I was remotely interested in. What this meant was that I didn't need to be in every conversation. Some things got directed to my hubby-to-be, and others things never reached me at all—my sisters were great filters!

I would be lying if I said it was easy to have the conversation. It wasn't. I was, at that time, talking to my mom almost every day, several times a day. But I wanted to talk to her and not think about getting married. I wanted to know how she was doing, and it's hard to have that conversation if we were talking about fabrics for my aso ebi. Holding the line gave me peace. Asking my sisters to be filters gave me support. Telling my momma and seeing how she worked within the boundaries also made me feel so very seen and loved. It let me know that my needs are valid and would be respected. It also helped me feel more confident in how I get to show up in the world and be received.

Holding the Line

Daily practices you can implement are fairly simple. Simple, not easy. Sometimes what you do on the daily can feel monotonous, but when you are just starting out in strengthening those boundaries, it can be helpful just the same. Here are three daily habits you can get into to help hold the lines on your boundaries.

1. **You can set the tone.** What are your intentions for your day? What goals do you have? (Please make those reasonable. There are twenty-four hours in a day, but every moment doesn't need to be goal focused.) What time can you protect in your schedule to make room for the goals you want to accomplish?
2. **Reflect, my friend.** I know. I keep telling you to reflect. But I keep saying it because I *mean* it. Grab a notebook and consider what went well or not so well in your day. Consider where your

boundaries were not well enforced or where they were ignored by the folk around you. What can you do differently next time? Are there conversations you need to have?

3. **Establish morning and nighttime routines.** Having a routine for waking up and winding down gives you more space to reflect. Not to mention it gives an opportunity for you to start your day with yourself intentionally and to end it with yourself with that same intention.

NICE VERSUS KIND

Within boundaries there is a space where we must examine if we are being nice (merely performing the niceties) or if we are being *kind*. Niceness is a performance of whatever societal expectations are placed at any given moment on you—often based on your gender expression, race, etc. You have to do certain things to be seen as a "nice person" or as a superficially "good person." I say *superficially* because folk don't need to know you to make this assessment; they just need to see the performance where you do what is expected based on how you present yourself in the space. Kindness, on the other hand, is steeped in what you know about yourself and moving more toward an authentic expression of that self in a way that is still appropriate for the venue. While niceness might be saying yes to something you don't want to do (even if that something brings up feelings of resentment, anger, or frustration), kindness is saying no because you don't deserve to feel like shit and you want to make sure they have the time and space to find the right person to do whatever has been asked.

Now when it comes to power, folk in positions of power certainly expect people who are trying to be "in their good graces" to perform niceties, particularly as deference in them. Now back in the day (pre-COVID, when money was looking a little different), I had an opportunity to go to Disney World and Universal Studios. Now, I don't know which park I was in, but I know I was having the greatest of times—a whole Harry Potter Head here and a girl who grew up on every damn Disney movie. Anyway, I am walking toward the middle but still firmly on the right side of the walkway, because we all know it works a little bit like road traffic. But there was a large white family coming, and they decided to spread out and were walking well over the invisible line of demarcation. I will admit that I was having an obstinate moment; I decided that for that day, I was not going to make room for someone who was decidedly not paying attention to their surroundings or reading the damn room. Well, this white woman walked full on into my chest. It wasn't enough that she was expecting that I would show her deference and move. She knew she was wrong—on the wrong side of the walkway and wrong for expecting my performance of a "Nice Negro Girl," but instead of contrition she decided to call me a bitch.

Let's start here: I know I wasn't right, but I also wasn't wrong. A boundary is the thing that *you* will or will not do. In this case, I decided that I would not be stepping off sidewalks or doing the little jig that can happen when you are trying to accommodate those who are allowed to take up space. This was me practicing taking up space, too. I did not move; that was my boundary.

My boundary cannot be that she will not call me names. Why? Because I cannot control her. I can't make her not call me a bitch; I can only question her decision to do so and/or remove myself from the situation.

The delusion of white supremacy requires that we bend to its "boundaries." Except that what is required are rules for us to follow, which is not the same thing as a boundary. A boundary is what you will do, how you will respond, not how you require others to behave, which is a rule of engagement, as it were. In this case, Black people become smaller because white people want to take up more space. Women become quieter because the patriarchy only makes room for male voices. When it comes to upholding our boundaries, we often make them malleable by trying to play niceties with others, which means our boundaries become negotiable. We negotiate our needs mentally, emotionally, financially, physically, in space, etc., in order to show deference to someone. If it doesn't feel good, it might be time for a change.

Remembering the following tips can help you hold the line:

You don't owe your parents

You don't have to forfeit the life you want—the life that pleases you—in order to fulfill the desires of your parents. You are their child, not their property. Your life need not be lived to only make them happy. Parents who are able to respect you and see you as an autonomous being, separate from them, will be sad to watch you leave their values and desires behind, but they will also be proud to see the person you become. If they can't do that, consider boundaries you may need to implement in order to maintain your mental and emotional well-being.

Your job is not everyone's happiness

This has been said time and time again, and it needs saying once more: if you make the happiness and contentment of everyone else your top priority, it means that you are NOT a priority. The people you're prioritizing will still be thinking of themselves and how *you* can help or serve *them*. And you, too, will be thinking about them and how you can serve them. It isn't conducive to knowing more about you and then meeting the need that your mind and body supply for you. Sometimes people will be saddened, upset, or even angry that we have boundaries—but it's often because *they* don't have them. Try not to take their feelings personally; it's not really about you; it's about them. It's about what access to your resources—body, brain, etc.—means for them and how it supports them. When we say no, we aren't saying it *to them* as much as we are saying it *for us*. If you don't protect your peace, there is no guarantee that the folk in your life are going to work on it in any significant way. If someone has to be sad, angry, or upset, don't choose for it to be you. Even if you choose your wellness and contentment, they still get to choose if they are gonna be angry and sour or if they are gonna find the good in your setting and maintaining your boundary.

Prioritize your shit versus their shit

Someone else's emergency is not your urgency. What my neighbor needs is not my job to supply. Remember there is your shit, and then there is other people's shit. If you take ownership of other people's stuff, you will feel responsible and obligated to constantly do for them. But if you can remember they are not you and you are not them, then you get to own your shit and they get to own theirs. Yes, you can be in community together, but it doesn't require you to take their shit on or in as your own.

If you treat time like money, you might say no to more shit

Consider your twenty-four hours. Consider what you need and want to get done, the time you will take for pleasure, rest, bonding, work, taking care of your body, etc., and then see how much time you have left. Now that you have subtracted all your wants and needs from your day, the rest is what's left to spend on other people. If you are giving time to someone or something else, it's time that is reallocated from you. This can help you be wiser about what you're saying yes to and making sure it's in alignment with your values, goals, and the pleasure-filled life you are working to build.

Boundaries: A Community Service

Because we are in an individualistic society, we often think of boundary setting as a thing we do for ourselves and for only our benefit. We don't often think of it as a display of good community behavior, a service. If you have not heard it, let me be the first to tell you: having boundaries is good for the collective, *and* it is great for you, too!

☕ *TEA TIME*

In late 2021, my family decided we would take a huge, all-out family vacation to Costa Rica. When I say *all-out,* I don't just mean the immediate family. Naw. My maternal aunt and uncle, and the cousins were coming, too. All in all, there were about fourteen of us. My sister and cousin found the spot we would stay in. Everyone looked into activities to do. Flight costs were researched, and we estimated the cost per person and put everyone on a payment plan for a year. In December 2023, the plans were set and paid for, and Costa Rica was calling our names! The crew in the DMV headed to the airport early, scoped out seats, and were waiting for the flight. I have flight anxiety these days, so, for me, beyond hand-holding and possible meds, I knew I needed snacks. My youngest sister and I headed to buy snacks for anyone who didn't wanna get up. While looking at the shelf of snacks, a woman came up behind me and told me my hair was beautiful, which I know it is. It was fantastically blue with purple highlights in spring twists that just beg to be photographed and touched. However, I ain't beg no one and this woman decided to put her hands in my hair without consent, just the same. I whipped around and asked, "Are you touching me?" She immediately dropped her hands and apologized.

The social contract in America says that Black people and women are up for grabs, literally, especially when someone feels tempted. The temptation, of course, is nothing more than thinly veiled audacious entitlement. Men who feel tempted are vindicated in their boldness to touch women they do not know on the streets. White folk are vindicated in their audacity to touch Black folk and folk of color because they were attracted to some feature or because something about them is unfamiliar. Questioning or rejecting male or white "compliments" and comments about your person are seen as an inability to "take a compliment" or come with the tag of being "mean" or a "bitch." You are supposed to be flattered by men who want to fuck you or by white women who desire to pet you.

However, we are changing the terms of the social contract so that it is no longer steeped in delusional supremacy culture, where someone can believe they have access to your body simply because you are taking up space in a public place. In my asking this white woman if she was touching me, it let her know that she has no right to touch me without my consent (which she was never going to get; I am not, after all, in a petting zoo), and it also showed my sister, who saw the exchange, that it is also okay for her to NOT allow someone to touch her.

So, when we have and hold the line of our boundaries, there are a couple of ideas we are adding to the zeitgeist:

We, as Black folk, as women, are allowed to protect ourselves, mentally, emotionally, physically, financially, socially, etc., by setting limits and saying no to those who we come in contact with.

We teach the people we hold boundaries with that they, too, are allowed to have boundaries that protect them and that we will respect those boundaries.

We teach people how to treat us, and, over time, how to accept and maybe find the joy in hearing the no. Because quiet as it's kept, some of us have no boundaries and then we expect everyone around us to also have no boundaries. As such, we get offended when they do.

BETTER BOUNDARY-BUILDING RESOURCES

→ *Set Boundaries, Find Peace* by Nedra Glover Tawwab
→ *Boundaries* by Dr. Henry Cloud and Dr. John Townsend
→ *Boundaries in Marriage* by Dr. Henry Cloud and Dr. John Townsend
→ *The Four Agreements* by Don Miguel Ruiz
→ *#RelationshipGoals Guide* by me, Dr. Donna Oriowo

You can find these books wherever you buy books, except the Relationships Goals Guide. Follow the QR code below to download the guide at the resource website for this book!

CHAPTER 7

Self-Talk *Is* Communication

Back when I was engaged and trying to live my best life during a whole-assed global panini, my friends flew me out to NOLA so that I could have my bachelorette party. Now I am a low-key kinda girl, which means that I wanted to simply spend time with them—and in the company of some great food. Anyway, we were sitting in our Airbnb's living room and one of my good girlfriends said something like, "I am so fucking dumb," in reference to herself. I ain't never been so quick with a comeback. I told her she needed to watch her mouth, talking to my friend like she crazy. With love, I reminded her that if I made a similar mistake, she would never tell me I was dumb. She would never say that shit to her kids, so I asked her why it was okay to admonish herself in that way.

This, my dear reader, is why we got to talk about our self-talk. When it comes to self-talk, we have to remember this: self-talk actually *is* communication! And considering the ways that many of us speak to ourselves, it's apparent that we need someone to yoke us up, with love, and remind us to WATCH. OUR. MOUTHS! Quiet as it's kept, we are constantly in communication with ourselves—thinking about our abilities, evaluating ourselves, and considering the things we should have done better or not fucked up in the first place. While we are in a space of wanting to improve and do better, being in a space where we're consistently and constantly chastising, admonishing, and belittling ourselves to the point where we make ourselves feel like shit is *not it*. So, let's talk about the five love languages and see if we can find new ways to talk to ourselves that better support our self-esteem.

Five Languages for Self-Love

When it comes to love languages, we have heard that there are five, though I think it depends on who you are talking to. For the purposes of this book, we will be referring to the five love languages as presented in *The 5 Love Languages: The Secret to Love that Lasts* by Gary Chapman. In his book, Chapman presents the following love languages:

1. Physical touch
2. Receiving gifts
3. Quality time
4. Acts of service
5. Words of affirmation

Now, if you are anything like me, you are reading this list and thinking, "Um… ma'am, four of these 'languages' don't say anything. How is this supposed to help my self-talk?" You would be right. I would be looking at me strange, too. But here is the thing, I am not just talking about how you *speak* to yourself; I'm talking about how you communicate, as a whole, with yourself. I think that we often get too caught up in what is *said*. We don't spend enough time remembering that words are only a small portion of communicating; the rest is in the tone we use, the way that the words are said, the way that information is presented, and the way that our bodies are moving with it. Just because there are no words does not mean that there is no communication. Besides, TALK IS CHEAP! It doesn't mean that it is not expensive to our psyche and impacts how we move, but it does mean that we have to make sure that (self-)talk matches that walk. Getting into alignment can also be helpful in getting the blueprints for your self-concept and using it to build your self-esteem. So, I want to make sure that we start here, because when it gets to a place of moving into affirmations and making sure that we're saying kind things to ourselves, we have to remember that doing things is a form of communication that we are going to have to work on, too.

A Side Note on Non-Verbal Communication

Seven percent. Just seven percent of communication is verbal, as in the words you use to say something.[1] That means that ninety-three percent of communication has to be accounted for by something else. When I say self-talk is communication, I am really only talking about that seven percent. But if we are gonna get to one hundred percent, then we have to account for how we practice the other ninety-three percent of communication.

☕ TEA TIME

On that note, let's look at *The Bodyguard*. A lil tea time about your girl: I am *obsessed* with this movie...judge your mama. Whitney Houston was singing, Kevin Costner was acting, and I am finally old enough to understand the story. Now I know the movie is from 1992, but I have been watching it since then. Get on YouTube and search for the scene that happens after Whitney sings "Queen of the Night" at the club. Kevin Costner, the bodyguard, and Mike Starr, personal security, have a whole-assed conversation in Whitney's kitchen with *no words exchanged* till the end. Now when you watch it, there is no way you can tell me that was not a whole-assed beautiful conversation about boundaries and expectations. The closing of that conversation lives rent free in my head: "I don't want to talk about this again." HA!

In this scene, much was said without words. The same thing goes for how we communicate with ourselves. If you want to communicate about how much you like yourself, respect yourself, and both display and feel your self-esteem like a warm blanket on a cold night, affirm that shit with your actions. Stop telling folks that you love yourself, like yourself, respect yourself, etc., when there's no evidence to support it. Maybe you are using your words to get you on the way, but like I said, talk is cheap. Would you even believe you? Be real. Because if you talk shit about yourself all damn day to any Tom, Dick, or Harry who will listen, then not only do they know where you stand, so do you. I said what I said. If you want to show people you like yourself, if you want to communicate to others (or to yourself) that you like yourself, then you need to hold yourself in the highest of esteem and live your life in such a way where you never have to open your mouth because your ninety-three percent is communicating it all.

This is not a fake-it-'til-you-make-it mantra; it's moving with the intentionality of treating yourself with respect, kindness, and care. It might mean dropping that fuckperson. It might mean looking for a new job. It might mean setting up that long overdue therapy appointment. It might mean celebrating the body you have with clothes you like that fit that body. It might mean eating foods that make you wiggle with joy in your seat. It may also mean telling your braider that she is gripping them edges just a touch too tight. And if she won't listen, drop her and find someone who will. Caring for yourself is not just an affirmation you say in the mirror, its finding and acting out the evidence that supports that care.

I'm saying that part of the communication for ourselves and others is showing, with our action, what caring for you looks like. To be clear: this is not to say that "if you don't show yourself care and love, that nobody else will," because you know I don't believe that. The right community can show us how to care for ourselves. The right community can also be a beautiful display of how we have already learned to care for others and be kind to them so we can figure out how to turn that love and kindness inward and let it continue to radiate outward. I am saying that you can teach people how to treat you better by treating yourself better. Don't just tell people; *show* them. Have a silent yet loud conversation with somebody while they/you eat a damn peach about boundaries and expectations. Say the thing with your words and say it again with your actions and choices. As Kevin Costner said: "I don't want to talk about this again."

PHYSICAL TOUCH

You are a person who deserves to be touched and to be touched with kindness. You do not have to endure pain to get beautiful results. Example: When it comes to our hair, I keep hearing people say, "I am tender headed." Which, for me, sounds like a self-chastisement that came from others. We say this instead of saying that we experience pain in ways that are different from others and thus require a different touch. If it stayed in the realm of our heart, perhaps I would feel differently, but it don't so I don't. The idea of us being strong and able to endure is made universal, from tresses to the relationships we have with others. We can take shit because "it's not that bad," "we have had worse," or because it's supposed to "teach us a lesson." It is an unfair ask for us to have to suffer in order to experience beauty with hair or in life. And it's also unnecessary because, like I said, we just need a different touch.

So, when it comes to physical touch, make sure that you are touching yourself in ways that are respectful of and good for you. A lack of pain does not mean there is a presence of pleasure. So don't just seek to not cause yourself pain; also try to seek out pleasure. That caring physical touch can show up in how you wash your hair. It could be in the way that you wash your face and body. Doing so with a gentle touch, relishing the way that you touch your body. Smoothing lotion into your skin, a nice caress. This can be a way of communicating to yourself, saying, *I care for me, and I care for me in such a way that I'm going to touch myself and ask others to touch me with hands that show caring, that show a sense of love* Now that physical touch can also move into a sexual touch. I am a girl who is all for masturbation, after all. And we're gonna get more into it in the next chapter.

✐ JOURNAL WORK

Consider some ways you can show self-care by way of physical touch. Write it down.

ACTS OF SERVICE

You deserve acts of service that help you to feel loved. This kind of love can open up your time, allowing you to experience more quality time with yourself where you aren't constantly doing things. Now you may not follow the suggestions I have here on a daily (or even a weekly) basis, but doing these things—especially when you have lots of things going on—can help relieve stress. While you can always perform an act of service for yourself, I am firmly on Team Get Some Help When You Want It.

☕ *TEA TIME*

I don't clean my house. I mean I do a preclean before the cleaning folk come, but I haven't had to actively clean my kitchen or bathroom in a long time. I added it to my budget as an act of self-care. When it came to laundry, a friend was so offended that I was spending my day off to do laundry that she sent me one hundred dollars to use a service.

Having someone clean your home is an act of service that you can give to yourself. It still gives you a clean home and you get to rest. Another is to send your clothes to a laundry service. If you have thirty dollars to spare, then you can get a laundry service. Pack up the clothes and allow somebody else to wash and fold them; you will be the one to simply put them away. These are simple small acts of service. Granted, these are acts of service that also require us to use money—and I don't know about you, but inflation got me looking at my wallet tryna figure out how to get that *Bodyguard* salary.

Here are other acts of service that are free, ninety-nine cents, or may cost you a pizza and a hug. You can try asking people in your life to help take something off your plate and allow them the space to do so. Remember that the "Fuck it, I'll do it" mentality is something that we are leaving in the past. Instead, we are getting help and knowing that we don't need to feel ashamed because of it. But you also don't need to moderate whether or not others are able to help you. We often consider what we think we know about someone's life and try to make a choice for them if they can help us. Stop it! Mind your business. Allow that person to tell you no so that you can stop telling yourself no in advance. Allow them to determine for themselves if they can. If you really want to help, you can ask them if they have the capacity, time, energy and space. If you get a no, then you know it's not about you, so don't take it personally. But when you get a yes, know that it is definitely for you! Other acts of service that are free(ish): fold and put away the laundry, organize your space, bake a treat for yourself, order groceries, massage your scalp, drink water, mind your business, masturbate, take a shower, massage lotion into your body. Make your list!

Being kind is also an act of service!

We have already talked about nice versus kind. But kindness is what we are aiming for, not being nice. Niceness is following a pre-scribed set of behaviors, observing the so-called "niceties" which can be dishonest in the way that we display ourselves. Niceness says that you should do the nice thing, even if it hurts you to make it happen. It doesn't have to be based in the truth of who you are, where you are, or your capacity. Niceness can take us away from ourselves and help us feel rather shitty.

Kindness, on the other hand, requires truth and knowledge of boundaries and of self because in kindness, you are setting boundaries according to what you know about yourself and what you need. You're trying to respect your space and you're trying to respect the space of others. When you are trying to be nice, you're often dismissing yourself in the process, which does not help you. Kindness is an act of service that gives you what you need and gives others the opportunity to figure some stuff out for themselves. A true win-win to support your self-esteem.

RECEIVING GIFTS

I don't know about you, but I like receiving gifts. While it can be a pain in the butt for my family during the holiday season when they are trying to figure out what to get me, I like to give myself gifts because it means I am not left wanting or waiting for someone to give me something I know I can give myself. It also means if they get me something I don't quite like or want, I am not left feeling disgruntled or disrespected. Baby, buy buy buy yourself a gift. Give yourself the gift of a clean home. Give yourself the gift of getting your hair done, buy new jewelry; get those glasses that you want. Buy some new underwear—whatever! All the gifts that you give yourself do not have to be top-notch, top-quality, frivolous sort of things. They can be things that you need that still feel like a gift-worthy act. On occasion, hit the gift wrap button at checkout. That way you can unwrap a gift from yourself. Can you promise yourself one gift a month? A treat you can wear, eat, or use? Try to budget for it every month because you also deserve nice things.

To date, my favorite gift to myself is a pair of over-the-ear noise-cancellation headphones. I can be sensitive to noise, and it helps me maintain my homeostasis. Another gift I cherish is my Appa AirPods case. You may not be able to buy happiness, but I was able to put a down payment on it for less than ten dollars.

(Yes, I am into *Avatar: The Last Airbender*. I really wanted my own sky bison.)

QUALITY TIME

Yes, we are always spending time with ourselves because we are in our own bodies. But the time we spend is not often *quality*. Many of us don't think about purposefully spending time with ourselves. Now this may not be for my introverts, because we def be spending time with ourselves; I am more talking about my extroverts. Spending quality time with yourself is a skill set that requires intentionality. For some of us, we may be alone, but that does not mean that we are intentional in how we are spending our alone time. We are not wooing ourselves. We are not taking ourselves on dates. We're simply sitting in our house while we binge Netflix and sit in a stupor.

I'm asking you to take intentional time to spend with yourself. Is there a place that you want to go? An experience you want to have? A restaurant where you want to taste the food? What are the things that you can do to make sure that you are spending intentional time with yourself? Quality time with yourself doesn't have to cost more money than what you are spending now.

I am a DMV girl. I like a free self-date in this area, and there are not many excuses. I've picked a Smithsonian Museum to visit, walked around downtown, and sat in a park. I also look up free and cheap things to do near me using social media and good ole Google! I take myself to the movies. I have also been known to take myself on trips out of the country, but those take a lil extra money. The point is to spend purposeful quality time with yourself. Are you a homebody who doesn't want to leave the house? Okay, quality time can look like reading books. It can look like intentionally watching a movie and curating a full moviegoing experience for yourself, making sure that you set up the snack stand the way you want it. It could be cooking yourself a meal, which also has a beautiful way of engaging your five senses. But quality time is just that: quality. It cannot be something that you slap together at the last minute with no thought. Think of it as taking yourself on a date. Maybe you can get lucky.

WORDS OF AFFIRMATION

And the most important seven percent is words of affirmation. I want to treat this love language like it's the most important, because how we talk to ourselves can also predicate how we show ourselves care. And like I said before, some of us have horrible self-talk. We talk to ourselves any old kind of way. I think we often forget that we are actually *listening*. We hear this self-talk, and we take it to heart. Sometimes the things we say become a self-fulfilling prophecy. If we talk shit about ourselves, we feel like shit and feel like we can't do shit. But if we can change it, who gon' check us, boo?

So, here's an exercise for you: I would like you to figure out the origin story of your self-talk. Too many things happen in community for me to believe that you came up with your regime of self-chastisement in a bubble. However, consider that although it may be your inner voice saying the words, you could be reading from a script given to you by a family member, a friend, society, etc. Think back and identify who said what. When did they say it? And also think about how it does and does not apply to you. Ask yourself, is it useful? Is what you're doing effective? Is it true? Would you say that shit to a friend? To a child? We are in the gentle parenting era, so I want you to try reparenting yourself with some gentleness, with kindness and find new ways to tell yourself things that don't require self-flagellation.

✐ JOURNAL WORK

What can you say to yourself instead of the negative self-talk you may use? Write it down. Practice saying it in the mirror.

A word on brutal honesty

No one has ever required brutality to be a side dish of the honesty that you want to serve them. Sometimes we are giving other people brutality because we have received brutality, not because they require it to learn. If you want to talk to people, and you want them to hear you and to appreciate what you are offering, then it may require you to actually consider your relationship with honesty that is brutal and may require you to consider why brutal honesty has become your bread and butter. Brutality, to me, in this sense, is a display of white supremacist tactics to elicit harm to get someone to yield to your desires. Honesty is hard enough; it does not require additional brutality. Telling people what you want them to hear can be done with kindness. That is not to say that sometimes it won't hurt; it is to say that unnecessary brutality is just violent and not as cute as we try to make it seem. So, if you have been known for your brutal honesty consider this: Why are you invested in being brutal? How does brutality add to your honesty? What is the goal in utilizing brutality? Is it effective? Is it helping your relationships?

Finally, we have arrived at manifestos and affirmations. Also known as ways we can actively speak kindness. One thing that my therapist had me do at the height of my anxiety was create a manifesto. A manifesto is a type of statement that speaks to your intentions, your views, and your motives. A written guiding purpose of how I'm living, how I would like to live, and a reminder of who I am and how I'll grow. While we cannot always know with one hundred percent accuracy how we will grow, grow we will. This is my manifesto. Feel free to use mine as a way to create your own:

I am free to be me and show up as such. I am open and honest with an unheard-of kindness. I am hopeful and planful. I am the sum of my parts and beyond it. I am that I am. I show up fully according to my needs and my commitment. I show up in the full might of the people who came before me. I show up as a beacon for Black girls who talk about pleasure. I show up for myself. I have space. I have support. I have that which I need, want, and desire to be as I am. I am God and God's blessed. I am covered. I am wisdom kissed. I am grown from Gaia and God. I am goddess and creator of my life. The world around me is cultivated and prepared for my success. Success is as I define it. Freedom, love, peace, happiness, and contentment are mine and entrenched in my growth as a perfectly imperfect creature. I am that I am and so much more.

I have my manifesto on my wall as a reminder of who I am and that the life I live is the one that I am choosing to create for myself.

✐ JOURNAL WORK

Write a manifesto for yourself. Feel free to use mine as an example.

An affirmation is a statement that you declare as true. Here are three of my favorite affirmations. Take some time-time to consider what you need to remember about yourself or what you need to speak into being and write some out for yourself. Think Issa Rae in *Insecure.* Your affirmations don't have to follow anyone's formula but your own. I will suggest this though: state what it is in the affirmative. Sometimes we default to what we don't want. The brain takes a bit longer to process the *don't.* Instead say what you want. So instead of "I don't want to be sad," consider what you actually want: "I am peaceful and content."

1. Pleasure is my birthright.
2. My success is guaranteed.
3. I show up for myself.

Relationships That Support Self-Talk

When it comes right down to it, we already know that self-esteem is built within the space of community. For us this means that our self-talk may also have started with the very communities that we are already embedded in, regardless of if we chose those communities. Sometimes the people in our lives are not kind. They say things to us that are not meant to help us or encourage us. Sometimes folk say things to be hurtful and harmful. And quite frankly, when someone is saying something that isn't constructive, it is likely you don't need to take their shit personally. What some folk say is more about them, and it says more about them than it does you. It doesn't mean don't evaluate and see if there is a nugget of truth in there for you, but be careful of barbed words. So, when it comes down to it, it might be time for you to evaluate your relationships and how you are feeling within them, and then figure which of those relationships need to continue as they have been or be dissolved.

Take a moment and think about your top five relationships. We're starting with five because it is often said that you are a compilation of the five people you spend the most time with. Their habits become your habits; their sayings become your sayings. I realized that I've been saying *bay-bay* And I got that from a friend. It just slipped its way into my lexicon. Another friend talks about being a badass a lot, since it's her brand; it too has slipped into my regular rotation. These are people whom I spend time with. These are people whom I love, whom I adore, whom I hold in high regard and esteem. But what I know is that they also hold me in high regard and esteem. And the way they talk to me has become reflected in the way that I talk to myself. I allow myself more space and grace because of how they speak to me, because they speak to me with love and gentleness because they are kind, not nice, and because they know that brutal honesty is lowbrow and lazy.

✐ JOURNAL WORK

Start evaluating your relationships: (1) write down your top five relationships, and then (2) write how you feel in each of those relationships. Consider the level of importance of that relationship.

1. With (name) _____, I feel
   _____in this relationship.

2. With (name) _____, I feel
   _____in this relationship.

3. With (name) _____, I feel
   _____in this relationship.

4. With (name) _____, I feel
   _____in this relationship.

5. With (name) _____, I feel
   _____in this relationship.

Now that you know who you're talking about and how you feel, consider how important that relationship is to you. Check out the resource website via this QR code for worksheets if you don't want to write up your own!

I've had clients who needed to spend some time evaluating friendships and previous romantic relationships that they're in, usually because they're looking to be in better romantic relationships.

I once had a client, let's call her Kenan, who was just a badass, right? She was amazing, smart, funny, and talented, but she felt like she was in a constant cycle where she never had any friends. It seemed as if no one wanted to *become* her friend or *stay* her friend. Well, she was in therapy because she felt that she and someone she called her friend were on their last leg. They were having hella problems—which is why she came to therapy, to preserve the friendship. In doing the work, she realized that her friend was a fan of brutal honesty, but she, Kenan, didn't need brutality or tough love to know that she was seen and cared for. She needed a friend who was going to talk to her differently, but she also needed to evaluate whether or not that was a friendship that she would even want or need to continue. So, I created a workbook for her, the *#RelationshipGoals Guide*. A simple evaluation of looking back in order to go forward.

Looking back first, what has the relationship been in the past? What was good about it? What was not good about it? How did it start? You know, getting into the origin story—so you can find your way back. The next step was to evaluate the present relationship. What does it feel like? What does it look like? And where do you want it to be? Because sometimes our honest truth is that we don't want it to be anywhere; we want it to stop. And that's okay. Because too many of us are holding onto relationships because they have longevity, even though they are corrosive. We don't want to be without friends, even ones that are not the best fit for us.

This is your moment to be able to evaluate what the relationship is, decide what needs to change, and recognize the responsibility and role that you have as a participant in said relationship. Relationships are not all good or all bad. They often are a mix. Evaluating your relationships gives you an opportunity to consider whether or not it is salvageable and what needs to happen. And for many of us, that means that we have to revisit Chapter 6 and get into being Bob the Builder of our boundaries. Because, sometimes, it's not that our relationships are bad; it's that our relationship with self has not been prioritized in any real way nor our needs communicated. So, you may need to evaluate the relationship that you have with yourself, your boundaries, and your needs, and then use them as a way to radiate outward and evaluate the relationships of the five people closest to you. Not physically close, but close mentally and emotionally. Are you getting the things that you need? Do you need to establish new boundaries? Continue to move outward from there, evaluating the relationships and determining how you would like to move forward, *if* you would like to move forward. When you do this, take the time to consider where your relationships are, and where you would like them to be. You are setting yourself up to have better communication with the folk in your life, who will help to model how you have communication with yourself. Who will speak to you with kindness.

CHAPTER 8

Body Mapping Self-Esteem

A quick FYI before you get started: this is a pretty short chapter. But with all its shortness, it is one that requires you to DO, not just read. Yeah, I am gonna talk about body mapping and all, but the goal here is that you actually do some body mapping.

Story Time

I once had a student at a school that I worked in who was bright, precocious, and apparently had anger issues. During our time together, we talked a lot about what she knew about herself, what she wanted other people to know about her, and how to communicate those pieces to those around her. Because, you see, children are often thought of as only being the extension of their parents and as having the job of being seen and not heard. And as a result, we act like they are not separate entities capable of their own thoughts and feelings that are worthy of expression. Well, this girl, she would get upset in a hot minute, particularly when she was feeling invisible and silenced, and she was known to throw a thing or two, including a fist.

In our time together, we body mapped. We wrote out what she knows about herself, the things that make her happy, the things that made her sad, the things that made her angry or frustrated. We wrote it out, then we mapped it out. What she discovered about herself changed the game! She discovered that when she was feeling particularly frustrated, she would feel it on her chest as pressure. But the action of it felt like it was in her hands. It showed up as the desire and need to throw things or slap somebody. When she got angry, her palms would itch. Discovering how her body reacted to feeling invisible and silenced gave us a chance to work on the undesirable behavior. She learned her emotions and the way those emotions were embodied, which helped her to learn when it was time to request an exit from her teachers and to call for help to process her emotions. To better support her, she told trusted teachers and adults about how her anger showed up in her body, and if she was scratching her palms in class, that she very likely needed a break, and they should ask her if she needed additional support.

This discovery, through knowing herself, communicating with others, and building a community of support meant that the safety issue of chairs flying across the room was largely mitigated. It meant she was better able to learn. It meant that her teachers could relax a bit. Paying attention to her body, her emotions, and learning and communicating her needs opened up a whole different set of tools for her use.

What Is Body Mapping?

Body mapping is pretty much exactly what it sounds like, friend. It is a tool that is often used in therapy to help a client map out emotions, trauma, pleasure, all kinds of things in order to better assist them with knowing what is going on in their body. Not to mention that it can help recreate or strengthen the mind–body connection. Because, let's be real, a lot of us are actually very disconnected (disembodied) from our bodies.

What I mean by *disembodied* is that you are not present in your body. You may also not feel safe in your body or feel in control of your body. The thing is, because we've been taught to be ashamed of our bodies (Black, fat, disabled, female bodies), we try to shy away from the feeling as best we can, which can mean being disembodied. For some of us, we are hoping to "fix" our bodies, which can mean trying to lose weight, adjust skin tone, or try to make our bodies do or be what it takes to be seen as acceptable in a society that doesn't appreciate Blackness or femaleness. Discipline and control become the name of the game.[1]

From the time we were in grade school, we were also taught to shut down the needs, desires, and pleasures of our bodies. I don't know about you, but back when I was in grade school, you had to ask permission to go use the bathroom. And your teachers could have told you no. Because as far as they're concerned, you don't really have to use the bathroom. It's almost like they think they're sharing your body with you. Girls and women are (mostly) passively taught that certain body functions are not ladylike, so we are holding in farts and being overly selective about when and where we can have a bowel movement. We've been told that we're supposed to eat at specific predetermined times a day for breakfast, lunch, and dinner, with maybe a couple of snacks in between, and that anything outside of those norms is a problem. I mean, far be it from me to tell you that this is a white supremacist colonial mindset on how you're supposed to regulate your body in order for someone else to make a buck, but, hey, that's not what you came here for.

What you came here for was to learn that there are numerous ways in which we've been taught to disconnect from and discipline our bodies. We don't feed ourselves when we're hungry, and we very rarely feed ourselves the things that we are actually craving, as though our bodies don't also know what we need. As though those cravings are not attached to something mental physical or other, but again, I digress. The point is, body mapping is a tool that we can use to recreate the disrupted mind-body connection so that we can know what is going on with us so that we can figure out solutions. What does body mapping require? An idea of your self-concept.

How Can We Use Body Mapping to Know Ourselves Better?

While using a feelings chart can help you identify what you feel and track those emotions over time, body mapping allows us to track our emotions within our bodies and pinpoint where in the body our emotions occur.

For me, this ends up being a conversation about thoughts, feelings, and behaviors—often conflated, but they are separate concepts nonetheless. I have seen that people often interchange thoughts with feelings and feelings with behaviors. In case I have not been clear, a feeling is not what you *think*, but rather what you *feel*. Feelings are the emotions that arise in you because of either what's going on in your surroundings or what's going on in your innerverse (inside yourself).

Thoughts are the things you think. They are not your feelings but what you might *think* about your feelings—or what you might think about your innerverse and the world around you. Both thoughts and feelings are needed and important, but again, they are not the same thing.

Behaviors are what you do. Behaviors can happen through choice, or they can be involuntary, but they are *not* your feelings. You didn't throw something because you were mad, you *chose* to throw something because you were *feeling* mad. Behaviors might feel like emotions, but feelings are not facts. The fact is that far too many of us allow anger or other emotions to drive the car, and then when it crashes, we say it was completely out of our control. You cannot control your emotions (you are intended to experience them), but you can control your thoughts, to an extent, and certainly you can control your behaviors.

What does this have to do with body mapping? It can be difficult to map your emotions or even your thought patterns if you won't recognize that there is a difference between these three concepts.

Body mapping is self-concept on a sheet of paper for you and others to see. What I mean is that a body map shows what you know about yourself. It shows that you understand how certain emotions impact your mind and body. It shows that you know what thoughts are sparked for you (though, not so much, since you probably won't be adding every thought you think here), and it shows that you understand how your body likes to move with all that input. It is hard to create a good and useful body map if you don't know anything about yourself, your feelings, your thoughts, or your behaviors.

Knowing what you feel and when you feel it is a start. However you have to go deeper, which can feel hella uncomfortable. The point is to take the time to sit in understanding of where in your body you feel those emotions.

Now beyond knowing where emotions reside and how they behave in your body generally, it can also be important to map where trauma lives in your body and how your body has been holding on to, reacting to, and living out that trauma. Additionally, as we've been talking about self-esteem, it's good to know where that lives in your body too. When you feel good about yourself. When you feel a sense of accomplishment. Where's that? If you get backhanded compliments, where does that live? If someone says something hurtful to you, where does that live? Because I'm willing to bet there's a lot of junk in some of those areas. Sometimes they live in our throats, our mouths, our backs, or our shoulders, and we carry the tension with us everywhere, feeling it more heavily in specific situations. There's a lot going on. And it is important for us to know what that thing is.

The hope is that by completing a body map, you are more aware of what is going on in your body. This gives you a better chance of figuring out what to do with it, communicating it with your tribe, and relieving the bodily pressure that builds up. With regard to self-esteem building, for many of us, we are disembodied—we are not present in our bodies. There are many reasons for it, but building a body map can help bring you back. This gives you the opportunity to be more present about what feels okay and what doesn't. It gives you the chance to learn more about yourself and to know how you feel.

You'll see in the tool section on the website (check it out using the QR code!) that you have access to not only a body map but also a video to further explain how to body map and what we are body mapping.

Now, you might be a book-book person. Meaning you are NOT going anywhere to get the tools. That's cool. I can walk you through it right here! Where do all the feelings live in your body? Grab some colored pencils, markers, crayons, colored pens, whatever, and map it here. Note where you feel each feeling and how those feelings show up. Be sure to fill in the key so you can remember what you mean, including the significance of colors. For example, if you have anger that bubbles red in your gut. The key should indicate that the color red represents anger, and you can draw bubbles in the stomach area. Examine yourself, then get to it!

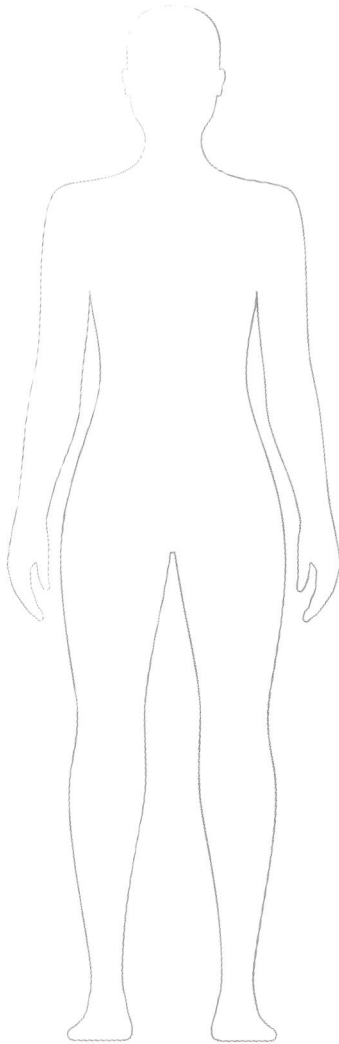

KEY

There have been multiple factors (friends, parents, etc.) we've talked about regarding self-esteem, but it can also be helpful to know how the people in our lives are related to our self-concept. And, of course, how it all shows up in our bodies. Ignoring an emotion is cute, but that doesn't mean it's not still showing up. Our bodies keep the score and act out when we don't have other ways to communicate or relieve it.

DON'T REPLACE YOUR SHIT WITH SOMEONE ELSE'S SHIT!

It's important to note that we shouldn't replace what we know about ourselves with someone else's construct of us. They don't know us any better. What I'm saying is this: Often we have parents who've known us our entire lives, or friends who've known us most of our lives, and they have fooled and deluded themselves into thinking that they know us better than we could ever know ourselves. They don't. In case you missed those words, I'm gonna say it again: **NO, THEY DON'T KNOW YOU BETTER THAN YOU KNOW YOURSELF.** They may *think* they know you better. They may think they understand what's going on with you because they've seen patterns in your behaviors. And it is not to say that they don't know a little something something, but they really only know what they see. They have had the honor of experiencing the you that you are when you are with them. They see you filtered through their own sense of self—talking and interpreting your actions and moods.

I am telling you this because when it comes to body mapping thoughts and feelings and noting corresponding behaviors, what the people who love you see about you doesn't supersede what *you* know. Now this does not mean that they don't see things about you that you don't see. Remember, the Johari window has the blind-self quadrant, so there is always something that people may see in you that you don't see in yourself. For example, if anyone would have asked me before Mr. BooThang and I moved in together, I would have told them that I love leftovers! Well, Mr. BooThang was the one who brought it to my attention that I do not like leftovers. He pointed out that I almost never ate them. It was something that he saw and knew to which I was just not privy. And yes, that blind-self quadrant also helps to construct our thoughts and feelings about others, even if we don't see it. The point is that even the you they experience is filtered through their own blind self. If they don't know themselves, they are likely to "see" something in you that actually has nothing to do with you and everything to do with what they don't know or understand about themselves–especially if they don't ask about their blind self.

Someone else's idea of you does not replace what you actually know, it is simply something to consider and ponder. You get to be honest with yourself and say if the thing someone else sees is actually true for you. This is why in my Johari window, I was able to give you an idea of what my blind self has. I've asked people what they see that I might not be aware of. I've had the, sometimes tough, conversations, people telling me that I'm arrogant, and we've had to have longer conversations about that. Am I arrogant or do you lack confidence? Am I a know-it-all, or do I simply not speak in question marks because I speak in definitive statements? I'm willing to be wrong, to learn, and to integrate new knowledge, but you have to actually tell me how I'm wrong. I'm not going to move with the assumption that I'm wrong at the beginning to assuage your feelings about the ways in which you might be right. The point is that we get caught up in ideas about what someone *thinks* they know about us, and as a result we remove ourselves from the reality of what we definitely know about us. We use other people's thoughts about us to not only obscure what we know about ourselves, but also as a way to define ourselves. And thus, we get into a cycle where we lie to ourselves using someone else's perspective. It doesn't make sense. So don't replace your shit with someone else's. This also means knowing that you cannot use their coping skills to make you feel better. Their body map cannot create yours. You are you, they are them, and you don't know what's going on in their body map until somebody explains it.

Let's Get Down to Business

At this point, you know a bit more about the whats and whys. But knowing what we are going to do and actually doing it are not the same thing. This section is about getting to work. So Part 1 of this work is just to write out the top ten emotions that you've experienced in the last week. What are your regular emotions? Check the feelings chart to get an idea, and remember a feelings chart is not exhaustive, it has *some* of the feels you can feel, not all of them.

Now that you know what you are feeling, take each emotion in hand and consider where you feel it in your body. What does it do in that part of your body? Does it pulse? Does it wave or does it flood? Does it flash and then go away? Note where it is in your body, how it shows up in your body, and then put it on your map. Choose a color that feels right for the emotion to you. Create the map in such a way that if someone were to pick it up, they would be able to say, "Oh, you hold anger in the color blue around your heart." It should be something that if you walked away from it for a year, you could go back and have a general idea and understanding of what it was. I don't know about you, but my memory be faulty, friend. So, consider creating a key.

Now that you have your emotions body map, there are some questions that I want you to consider when it comes to self-esteem and where it all lives in your body, specifically.

We talked about self-esteem being on a spectrum. Write down where on the spectrum you think your self-esteem is when you are at work, with friends, when you are with family, when you are with a lover, and when you are alone. You can do it on a scale from 1 to 10, where 1 is very low esteem, and 10 is very high or present esteem. The point here is that how you feel about yourself can vary with the company you keep.

✐ JOURNAL WORK

In your journal evaluate your self-esteem by giving yourself a score in a range from 1-10 for the following categories.
1 indicating low esteem, 10 indicating high esteem:

1. at work
2. with friends
3. with family
4. with lover(s)
5. when alone

Now that you have thought about and felt those answers, let's map them. What happens in your body when you're at work and you consider how you feel about yourself? What are the primary feelings that come up for you? What are the primary feelings that come up when you're with friends? When you're with your parents and family? What are the feelings that come up for you when you are with your lover? What about when you are alone?

PRO TIP: Sometimes it's hard to pinpoint how we feel about ourselves when we are with someone or doing something. So, consider how you feel immediately following being with that person or being at work. Do you feel happy? Is it just sort of glowing through you? Do you feel drained? Angry? Frustrated? Content? Like you wish a bitch would? Also consider how you feel just before you see this person or enter this setting. Are you preparing yourself for fuckery? Are you excited? Do you feel the need to change up pieces of yourself in order for you to have some peace when you're with them and when they are near? In what ways are you changing? We're mapping these feelings because they tell you how you feel about yourself in the presence of others. And whether or not those are feeling healthy for you.

Ultimately, body mapping can help you to spend some time in your feelings and body, so that you can get to know it, and in the end determine what you are going to do to keep your peace. This can help you to become the Bob the Builder of your boundaries. Part of it is knowing you so well that you can discuss that with others.

This is also a great time to use the self-talk that we discussed to help build that mind–body connection so that we can stop being disembodied from ourselves and depend on outside forces to help us feel good. Told you this was a short chapter. You got work to do.

Next chapter...mapping pleasure!

CHAPTER 9

Pursuit of Pleasure

Throughout my years as a therapist, I have met many women who have wanted to increase their self-esteem and heal from trauma they have experienced. Well, none more than Sharika. Sharika had a lot of trauma from her past, cumulated from various experiences in work, life, and the military's impact on her family. This brown-skinned woman was focused on healing from her past like it was a job—more than ten years in and out of therapy focused on trauma, anxiety, depression, and self-esteem.

While that work was very important and helpful, we really noticed a shift when we changed tactics. I couldn't be another therapist in her life focused only on the worst shit that ever happened to her, especially since she was tired of being in the muck of it all and wanted to start feeling better *now*. So, we took a different approach: we talked about pleasure. Instead of asking her about how she has been able to manage and move through all the pain in her life, I asked about her capacity for pleasure. Now, mind you, that question stumped her for a good month, but she sat in it and eventually realized that so much of her life and identity revolved around what she was able to endure, not what she *enjoyed*. When we focus on life's pleasures, it doesn't mean that we've stopped exploring the BS, but it does mean we aren't spending all our time there. So, when Sharika came to this realization, she started to see and experience herself beyond what she could endure. She started to learn and relearn other things about herself, and her relationship with herself and her self-esteem started to change. While she still had work to do regarding depression, anxiety, and PTSD, she said, "I feel like I can breathe again."

When I've told people that pleasure and the pursuit of pleasure can increase their self-esteem, a lot of people just sort of look at me sideways. So, I'm gonna say it again here: **When you are actively and purposely pursuing pleasure, you are also increasing your self-esteem.** Now you might be asking how that could be true, but if you take it back to Chapter 1, you will remember that I said, *self-concept informs our self-esteem*. The more you know about you, the more that you learn to like about you, understand about you, and take pleasure in, the more you will increase your self-esteem. So, when I tell you to pursue pleasure *on* purpose and *with* purpose, I'm telling you that doing so can actually increase your self-esteem.

Pleasure beyond Your Pants

Adult minds are nasty...and I love it! The problem is that when we hear the word *pleasure* so many of us immediately jump to how we get tangled in the sheets alone or partnered. This is sad, because it can limit the imagination on what is pleasurable and limit the ways we seek pleasure.

Sensuous or sensual pleasure is almost exactly what it sounds like. It's using your five senses—sight, smell, taste, hearing, and touch—to figure out what brings you pleasure and to create an environment of pleasure within you. It's about how we experience our bodies and how we lean into that pleasure. Because when we think *pleasure*, we usually *think sexual pleasure*, and don't do the work to separate the sensuous/sensual from the sexual, but the reality is that they are not the same thing. Sexual pleasure is (obviously) about sexual gratification and what feels good in a sexual sense. While sensuous pleasure can be part of that, sensuous pleasure alone is not inherently sexual. Sensuous and sensual pleasure can be as lovely as how you feel licking lavender honey from your finger, and licking that same honey from the neck of your lover. That is to say, there is a spectrum from the delightful that has nothing to do with being sexual to the delightful that is very much steeped in the sexual. To have more self-esteem, experiencing pleasure in both sensuous/sensual and sexual ways can be hella important and give us much needed space and opportunity to learn ourselves, no partner required!

When you are able to cultivate pleasure and feel comfortable with it in one area of your life, you are better equipped to experience it in other areas too. Here is a little of my business: one sense that I love to engage is hearing. There are beats and sounds that almost always bring me immense pleasure in the music I listen to. For example, there's a song called "Ocean Avenue" from the early 2000s, and I really just love the beginning of it every single time the beat drops...or rather becomes more robust. It just feels so refreshing. It makes me laugh a little, and it makes me feel so joyful. Same thing with Linkin Park and that song "Faint" or "Cold" by Maxwell. Just the sound of it, the way the horns come in, and his voice, whew!!! This is a song I blast so I can get a feel of those horns. Not to mention "Suavemente" by Elvis Crespo, and the beginning of "Unpredictable" by Jamie Foxx, which I start over and over again until I am satisfied!! Baby, I am a horn-hoe! It brings me joy when I hear it.

As for my other senses, I find immense pleasure in the beach. Going to the beach is a pleasure that engages all five of my senses, though a little less so for taste. I love the meeting of the sea, sand, sky, sun, and someone special to sit with. The feeling of sand between my toes, of the water rushing over my feet, the feel of the wind. The soothing sound of the ocean. This is something that brings me pleasure in a nonsexual way, but I know that it also gives my sexual self something to consider. Being able to learn this about myself and trying to pinpoint my why—as in why this experience is so delicious to me—means that I get the opportunity to learn about myself and give myself more of what I enjoy.

Taste is one of my favorite senses to indulge because for me it also involves touch, with texture. My taste sense is very food focused, but yours doesn't have to be. My hubby makes this dish from a cookbook called *Early Enough* that makes me wiggle in my seat and hum while I eat! Some of us don't eat with a sense of pleasure though; we eat per-functorily. We choose foods based on their nutritional value only and won't also look at the taste as a factor for mental/emotional/physical enjoyment. I mean, I guess I get it...not really, so to each their own, but I look for the pleasure in almost everything I am doing.

✐ JOURNAL WORK

Getting to the pleasure is your assignment! Take a moment to consider what it is that brings you joy and pleasure with regard to sights, smells, sounds, sensations, and tastes. What, from your senses, has brought you joy in the past? For me, it'd be my mama's jollof rice. A spicy Jamaican beef patty. Chicken with the perfect mumbo sauce. These things bring me joy. Clearly, I be in my stomach. Make a list of those sensuous pleasures. Don't lose this list; we will need it later.

The Benefits Package

We've already gotten into a whole definition of sensuous pleasure and explored some of my pleasure business, but have we talked about the benefits of pleasure? No, we haven't. Smh. Let's back into it.

There are lots of benefits to pleasure. Allow me to count the ways!

1. Pleasure can reduce the effects of stress and anxiety on the body, allowing you to feel more relaxed. And make no mistake, stress is a whole-assed killer! Black may not crack, but stress does kill.

2. Pleasure can increase dopamine and endorphins leaving you feeling happy, and well...it can also help reduce the feelings of depression.

3. Pleasure can help improve your quality of sleep and how long you're able to sleep—meaning you are better rested and maybe less grumpy.

4. Pleasure can help boost your immune system so your body is better at fighting off other folk's germs—and who doesn't want to be sick a lot less often?

5. Wanna have better circulation and keep the heart strong? Try pleasure. It works for that! Because pleasure helps with circulation, you can spend less on expensive face creams because baby girl will glow with health! We won't know who is more radiant, the sun or you.

6. Pleasure can reduce muscle tension and pain...probably because you are more relaxed.

7. Can't remember where you put your keys? Pleasure can help. Pleasure helps improve cognitive functioning and memory. Not only will you be able to learn things easier, but you will also be able to tell folk what happened on July 4, 1998, with no problem, while pulling all the receipts!

8. Pleasure can increase creativity and your ability to problem solve. Sounds like something your boss probably wants from you at work, and all you gotta do is employ some pleasure to get it? Sounds like a win!

9. Pleasure can improve your relationships with friends, family, and lovers! Meaning more intimacy (not just sexual).

10. Pleasure can improve symptoms related to anxiety and depression, so your mental health can improve, and you might be able to get off the therapist's couch.

11. Pleasure can also help with your digestive health and help you drop the kids off at the pool (to be clear, I mean *poop*) with more ease.

12. Pleasure can improve your sexual health and well-being. When we are seeking pleasure, we enjoy it more!

13. When you are pleasure filled, you can also more easily fill those lungs with air. You breathe better, which sparks even more health benefits!

14. Sexual pleasure through masturbation or sex can help you in these ways:

    a. Make menstrual cycles way less painful

    b. Help with that pelvic floor (which leads to stronger orgasms and to making sure you don't pee a little when you laugh)

    c. Lower that blood pressure

    d. Build your immune system

    e. Improve your self-esteem (goes with the book!)

    f. Increase your libido

    g. Help you get better sleep

    h. And get a good workout (WebMD says it counts as exercise!)

15. Pleasure in and of itself can also just help you feel happier, better, and more satisfied.

So, you might be looking at the list and thinking, "Ma'am, you got repeats here in number 4. Pay attention!" I did it on purpose, friend! Sexual pleasure added with your general pleasure is a double-your-pleasure, double-your-fun moment.

Ultimately, people who pursue pleasure are having a more pleasure-filled life instead of one that they feel the constant need to escape from.

✐ JOURNAL WORK

Take a moment to write down your definition of *pleasure*. What benefits have you seen in your life when you take the time to make pleasure a priority? What are the consequences when you don't?

Play Yourself

There is joy and innocence in play. I don't know about you, but I grew up playing freeze tag and hand games, jumping rope, riding bikes, and throwing in a little Nintendo every now and then for some razzle-dazzle. Some of us were doing the absolute most as children! We played for the sake of play. We played for our pleasure. And high-key, low-key, some of us played because our parents wanted us out of the house for a couple of hours. I grew up in a generation that was constantly being told, "You smell like outside," drinking out of a water hose, hanging out on the swings (and wanting to go over the top), and being present with our friends in the moment.

Everything was outside, and outside was where we wanted to be. But as we grow up, we do more inside things. Some of us can go days, especially when the sun sets early, without ever seeing the sun but through an office window. We stop being outside in the same way. We stop seeing being outside as everything we want. And suddenly we are divorced from play in favor of longer classroom times, and this removal from play and from being outside is seen as a rite of passage into "proper" adulthood.

When we think about play as adults we often think about sexual play, not just playing because it's fun and for the sake of pleasure.

Well, I'm here to tell you that in *my* house, we play. I visit my sisters and we roller-skate. We play with hula-hoops. We jump rope outside and we got those good ropes, too—since I am a real adult with enough money to buy things to play with. We play outside. Why? Well, it's not because I am trying to recapture my childhood. It's because I am trying to capture joy. I am trying to bottle pleasure. I want to see the stress lifted from the shoulders of my family members. I want the space to be silly and as unserious as I can be. I want my legs to remember the rhythm of double Dutch and to turn ropes often enough that I am never double handed. When I play, I not only feel a sense of pleasure, but also of peace and accomplishment.

The ways in which we play as adults don't have to look very different from the ways that we played when we were kids. We may have had less fear and way fewer responsibilities then, but now we have a better concept of consent and a more familiar relationship with our bodies, and we can ask outright whether or not somebody wants to play with us. You are not a person who is above play unless you decide that you are.

Play can be helpful in how we show up in our relationships, not just with others but also with ourselves. We can use play to heal emotional harms, help us develop and improve our social skills, learn to cooperate with others, and give us more space to open up for more intimate relationships. I may not have said it before (just kidding, I know I def did), but community is a huge part of developing a healthier sense of self-esteem. And play can help with that. Taking life so seriously all the time with work and familial obligations doesn't leave a lot of room for feeling good about yourself or your life. Not to mention that play and pleasure are revolutionary forms of resistance, like rest.

✍ JOURNAL WORK

Grab a friend and go play! Plan a game night. Buy some ropes, skates, or a hula-hoop. Schedule time in the next two weeks to play. When you're done with that, schedule another play-date in the next two weeks. Be sure to journal on how it was for you to play and what it's like to act like a parent scheduling a playdate.

Sexual Pleasure

Pleasure in general gets a fairly bad rap. It is something to be earned, not something to simply have. When it comes to sexual pleasure—both from a masturbatory practice and body sharing with lovers—now we *really* get into trouble. Sexual pleasure gets an even more salacious rap than just pleasure in general. What I mean is that on the one hand, when most of us think about plea-sure, this is what we jump to. We think about the ways in which we have been able to have sexual pleasure with ourselves and partners—granted, some of us are also thinking about the ways we become award-winning actors with the way we be faking it, but I digress.

As adults, sexual play becomes the only type of playtime and playdate that we know, and for me, that is very much part of the bad rap it gets. We inflate and center sexual pleasure, and conflate it like it's the only type of pleasure that is worth having when we become adults. Of course, the other part is the salaciousness and depravity that is supposedly uniquely associated with it. The judgment from church, family, and society if you appear to be enjoying sexual play too much or with too many partners. Women are taught that they must navigate the space between looking sexy and being ready for sex while still being aloof about it to maintain a good marriageable girl image. We are going to get more into it and will be covering both the self-pleasuring and the shared pleasure where it comes to sexual pleasure.

FRISKY FINGERS

Frisky fingers can help us move from feeling ourselves to *feeling ourselves!* So, masturbation is the act of touching yourself. And there are so many benefits. So many, in fact, that I created the *30 Day Masturbation Guide* to explore these benefits and help folk heal from the associated guilt and shame. The point is that when it comes to pleasure, and masturbation specifically, many of us have *a lot* of hang-ups. We have a whole Tabernacle Choir telling us about our place in hell and why sex makes us a bad person, all while governments try to keep the pleasures of sex a secret by not having countrywide, accurate, comprehensive sex ed. It's just one of the things you are not supposed to talk about, but when it's time to produce children, the grandparents-to-be want like three of them. Beyond the orgasms and babies to be made, I end up right back at this question: **WHAT IS YOUR CAPACITY FOR PLEASURE?** And this is a difficult question for people to answer, because many of us have been raised on our capacity to endure pain, whether that pain is from dealing with harsh loved ones, enduring racist and sexist work culture, dealing with partners who don't quite love us enough or the way we need, or friends who feel more like competition than companions. Whatever it is, we've been taught how to deal with pain, how to press on. How to ignore the hurtful parts so we can enjoy some of the albeit paltry benefits. To be in pleasure is something completely different.

And while there are many benefits to a masturbatory and shared sexual practice—ranging from lower blood pressure to exercise to mindfulness, and all the benefits that come with these—there is also harm that has already been done because of what church, society, and family have taught us about sex, mostly covertly, about who's going to hell, who's deserving, and who is not, all based on the level of engaged sexual activity. Those things can get in the way of building a successful practice. Of being able to reap the benefits of a pleasure practice, sexual or not.

Another benefit of masturbation is that it is actually a mindfulness practice. Having a mindfulness practice is really great for setting your mind at ease, bringing you to the present moment, and allowing you space to let things go and destress. You may now be wondering: "Wait, how is masturbation a mindfulness practice?" I am glad you asked! Because when you are masturbating, you are thinking about what brings you pleasure in that moment; sometimes it has no words. It's all feelings and sensations. Sometimes you may be fantasizing. Regardless, when you are masturbating, your mind and your body are often of one accord.

Masturbation can also help improve your communication skills! I know that it seems off, but the point is that when you masturbate and you know your body, it is easier to teach your sexual partners what you like and don't like so that they're able to perform to the level that you desire (instead of you just enduring what they give you). It can also help, of course, in your own learning curve; the more you know about your body, the more you're able to give it what it actually likes. Give more pleasure to yourself as opposed to enduring things that you don't enjoy.

This is just the tip...of the iceberg (*Didja think I was gonna write something else?*) when it comes to the benefits of masturbation. There are so many more benefits that we miss out on if we don't practice masturbation—and that's largely because we have been taught to feel shame around sexual pleasure in general, and around building a masturbatory practice, specifically. The shame we feel about sexual pleasure translates into how we feel about our bodies. Then the shame we generally feel about our bodies, how they look, function, etc., shows up in how we relate to others with our bodies, how we relate to ourselves with regard to our bodies, and ultimately, how we feel about ourselves.

IS IT UGLY OR UNFAMILIAR?

When it comes to what we consider to be beautiful or ugly, sometimes the difference is in what we're familiar with and what we're not. We have been taught certain people are ugly, certain bodies are ugly, certain skin tones are ugly. Meanwhile, if you saw more of those differences in appearance, if you saw the variations in them, if you saw the way people take pleasure and joy in them, you might think and feel differently. You could even think they're beautiful. Because our pleasure scripts are often written by other people and then carried out, unexamined, by us, we simply perpetuate the status quo. If you want to change your relationship with pleasure, with what you believe is great about your body, you have to look at it and engage with it a little bit more. Learn to appreciate certain pieces of it. See it for what it is, instead of always seeing for what it's not.

Pleasure ain't no joke, friend. It's not something to sneeze at. It's not something to scoff at. It's not something to doubt the importance of. Because it could be a priority. Hell, I'll say it: it *should* be a priority. If the poison is that we live for others—and the impact of that is destruction for our mental and emotional well-being— then the remedy is pleasure that centers the self.

So, what can you do? How do we get past the shame to reap the benefits of pleasure? You can get acquainted with your body, but it may require you to answer these questions first:

→ What did you learn about masturbation when you were growing up from the people in your life and from the media?

→ How would you characterize your feelings and attitudes about masturbation?

→ In what ways has racism and sexism impacted your experience of pleasure, including shared pleasure and masturbation?

→ In what ways have colorism, texturism, and featurism impacted your masturbatory and self-pleasure experiences?

And here's a hard question for you:

→ Do you believe that you are worthy of experiencing pleasure? Or do you believe that pain and suffering will build your character and make you the most defined version of yourself? A.k.a.: What is your capacity? For pleasure? And how have you found it?

A quick word on body sharing

When it comes to shared sexual experiences, everything that has already been said applies here, too. But now we add in body count culture, and you have a whole other thing that gets in the way of experiencing pleasure, because we are placing limits. If no one has told you, allow me to be one the of the first:

Promiscuity ain't nothing but deep sexual research with enough partners to know yourself, what you like, and what brings you sexual pleasure. Most people don't actually lack discernment in who they are sleeping with; we just act like they do so we can feel superior to them in our own sexual choices—which leave so many of us feeling bereft and deprived. This is a form of respectability politics by way of sexuality. And what we know is that respectability politics, no matter which way you spin it, have never been beneficial to the person who was trying to adhere to them.

But you, along with your partner(s), have the added benefit of your bodily knowledge and the pleasure map that you create.

SEXUAL PLEASURE FEELING STUNTED?

Drink water. Eat a Snickers. You're not you when you're hungry. Y'all, sometimes the body is not responding the way that you want your body to respond for a very simple reason: you're dehydrated. I said it. This is something that my good girlfriend Goody Howard talks about quite a bit—that we will be underfed and underwatered, yet we will still be demanding the absolute most from our bodies. In those instances, we're wanting the most while giving the least. Give to yourself; nourish your body. The pleasures that you want to partake in requires you to take care of your body. So, eat and drink with regularity.

Pleasure Mapping

Creating a pleasure map actually requires you to make two separate maps: one nonsexual and one that's all about sexual pleasure. During this process, the thing to keep in mind is that this is a living map. What that means is that the things you like and enjoy will change throughout your life, so your map will change, too. All you have to do is add things as you come across them, and remove things that are no longer pleasurable.

First, let's start with the nonsexual map. Remember those five senses that we talked about earlier, and the things that bring you joy through them? It is time to use those to create a pleasure map.

Consider where that joy lives in your body. How it shows up. As you think of it, be sure to add it to your body map. Think about what it feels like when you place a chocolate square on your tongue, when you hear that song, when you get that cozy blanket or those fuzzy socks, when you see that thing that just makes you sigh a little. Now map it out. What are the things that bring you pleasure?

Sexual Pleasure Mapping

Next, create your sexual pleasure map. Consider what your masturbatory practice has been. How do you like your body to be touched? Where do you like your body to be touched? Where do you like light touches versus deep strokes? Where do you like butterfly kisses? Where do you want almost touches? For far too many of us we see our sexual organs, pelvic areas, vaginas and vulvas, breasts, and anuses, as our main sources of sexual pleasure, but the entire body is your playground. So, when you think about what brings you pleasure, think about the entire body as a playground. Consider the ways in which your nonsexual pleasure map intersects with your sexual pleasure map. In what ways are they the same? In what ways are they different?

After both maps are created and you can see your good work, let this be a conversation starter that you have with every partner about what you like and what you don't like. And anyone who would have the gall to tell you that having a pleasure map and knowing your body means that you are promiscuous, tell them I said to mind they no-pleasure-having-assed business!

PLEASURE MAP

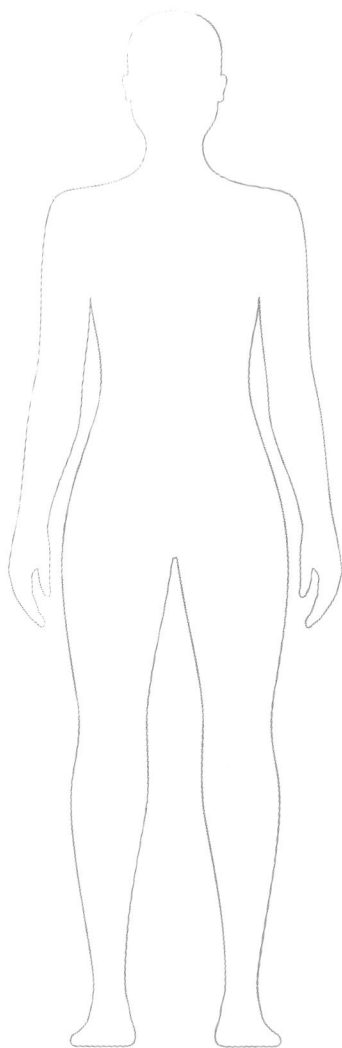

KEY

SEXUAL
PLEASURE MAP

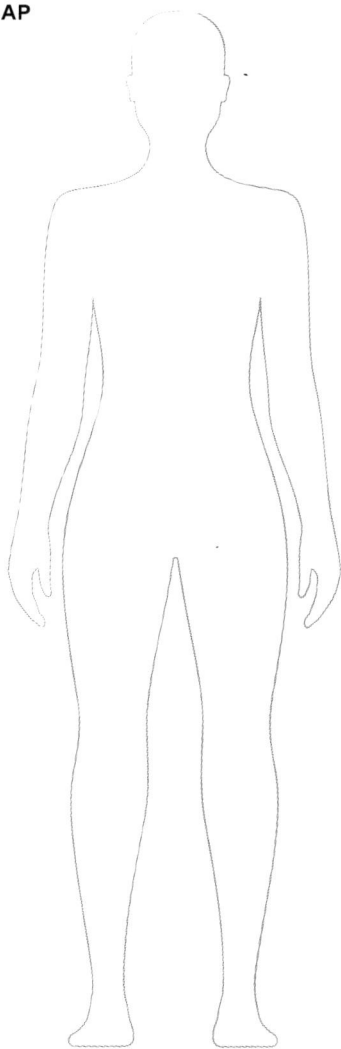

KEY

CHAPTER 10

BE LITerate

The world around us is constantly sending us messages. These messages are delivered through commercials, movies, TV shows, magazines, social media and all its shenanigans, and more, and they tell us about our place and value in the world fairly overtly, but mostly covertly. It's very rare that one of these entities will outright tell you that you are too ugly, too dark, too fat, too undesirable as you are. No, the message is way more insidious than that. They *imply* that you're ugly. They imply that you are too fat, too loud, too bold, too whatever. Then they suggest ways for you to fix it with creams, pills, clothes, diets, and more.

There is a quote by Charles Baudelaire that says, "The greatest trick the Devil ever pulled was convincing the world he doesn't exist." Now turn *Devil* into *devils* which for me is moving from the big scary thing to the smaller evils of the world, and I am in full agreement with the quote. A message that is said aloud is easier to fight against. When tyranny and bullshit are loud and in your face, you know you are the target, and you're able to get your lick back. You are able to fight against it. You are able to point out what is wrong and why.

When it comes to the battle for your self-esteem, the "enemy" is much less obvious. They don't outright say you're ugly, but they will show you who is cute. They don't tell you that you're not the right kind of Black, but they will give you an example of the type of Black you should be in order to be accepted.

They have hidden these messages in pretty prose and use beautiful actors to convey them: "You are not worthy," "Something is wrong with you," "You must change yourself to become _____." Fill in the blank "beautiful," "intelligent," "worthy of marriage," etc. There is an insidiousness to how the world tells us we are not okay or not right. The avenues for our entertainment and information have become fraught with little devils telling us something about us is wrong or broken, while simultaneously convincing us that their message is different, and that the devil they are simply doesn't exist. This is what requires us to have our wits about us and our eyes wide-open to make sure that we can not only see what's going on, but so that we understand the unstated messages and can chart a course of action that best serves us.

Reorganizing around Social Media

There's this video on social media that likes to circle back around every now and then; it's of this beautiful young Black girl, maybe between the ages of five and seven. In the video, she is getting her hair done, and she says, so matter-of-fact, with the lusciousness of her dark skin and the upward reaching of her kinky, coily hair, that she is ugly. The adults in the room say, "Don't say that." They tell her how beautiful she is, and the little girl just starts bawling. Now here's the thing, judging by the adults' reactions, it seems clear that no one at home told her that she was ugly. But somewhere along the way she picked up on the message that her skin tone, and likely her hair texture, bar her from being beautiful. She is a Black girl who likely watches TV, and TV does not praise little Black girls. Maybe someone, somewhere outright called her ugly, but the more likely scenario is that she received this message covertly. These covert messages, which many Black girls understand by the time that they are five years old, say that they are not and cannot be beautiful if their skin is dark and their hair is nappy. How will that girl grow up? What might she one day understand about what was said and what was not?

Let me lay a different example on you. I had a client who once upon a time told me that she was dark, fat, and nappy and asked me who the fuck was going to want to be with her. And while doing work with this client, what we realized is that no one ever outright told her that she was ugly in her family. They talked about how she was capable, how she was smart. They told her that she was going to be the one to help uplift her siblings and be a great support to them. They told her that she was going to rock it out academically and then be a rich bitch able to take care of her siblings and her mama. But notice what wasn't said: they never said that she was beautiful.

While no one explicitly told her that she was ugly, she got

the message: her job was to achieve so she could be a mule for her family. Her job was to give to her family. Her job was to use her body, her intelligence, then eventually her money, time, and energy to make sure that her siblings and her mama were taken care of. She watched her mom fawn over light-skinned cousins, telling them how gorgeous they were and talking about their prospects for romantic partnership. And yes, telling them that they are smart and capable, too. In private conversations, her mom would also disparage certain light-skinned people for acting like they are all of that, for being uppity and looking down their noses. But the message was clear to my client. She could never be "all that" because she wasn't light enough to be pretty. She didn't have the type of hair that her mother would fawn over. She didn't have her mother's or her family's attention, except for the excitement they had about what they could get from her. This is part of how colorism often works. Dark-skinned people are seen and treated as labor for light-skinned people, to be the mules.

And now I'm gonna feed it back into fiction. We talked earlier about the story of the little pig-faced girl from that movie *Penelope*. Penelope's mother never outright told her she was ugly, but Penelope got the fucking point. She got the point by the way her mother hid her, kept her in the house, and kept trying to find somebody (anybody) to tell her that they loved her. She got the message that she was unlikable and unlovable in her current form and that that form would need to change in order for her to live the life that she (and mostly her mother) deserves. That she would have access to the life her money, status, and white skin afforded her.

The point is this: the world around us is constantly giving us messages; it is constantly telling us who is worthy and what makes that person worthy without ever actually saying a thing. We know that dark-skinned women are often not the love interests in movies. We know that dark-skinned women are not often seen as someone to love but rather as someone to fuck. We see that light-skinned and white-skinned women are the love interests, especially if they're thin and have long wavy hair, light-colored eyes, and maybe even a dusting of freckles. They are still dehumanized and set as a prize for the "worthy" male companion, whose only accomplishment is noticing her and coveting her. Theirs is a story that is tied to how they look. Theirs is a story tied to the type of person that is considered good, righteous, deserving, loving, worthy of having self-esteem. We have discussed this, but we have to be woke. We need to be enthusiastically LITerate. We have to understand what we're seeing so that we don't inadvertently continue to digest messages that disparage our humanity.

Outta Pocket and Outta Context

One thing about social media is that it is as fun as it is addictive. These algorithms be algorithm-ing, and, baby, they are made to keep you on the app. And that's the thing that we have to understand. Social media, like any other type of media, is meant to be consumed. And all of these apps are in competition with one another. They are trying to outdo each other. They're trying to keep eyes on the app because that's how they make money, by learning about you and then selling your data to the folk who wanna sell more things to you. Understanding and remembering the goal of social media means that we are better equipped to understand where we stand with it. And that means that we have to understand social media headlines and clickbait, which I'm now thinking of more as outrage bait.

Falling into the hole of social media can leave a hole in your day—a gap of time that you just wonder where it went. But time isn't the only thing that's lost on social media; there is also a loss of understanding and a loss of energy. It sucks and takes from us. It takes our time, our attention, and our energy as it continually feeds us the same messaging on repeat. This is especially true for apps like TikTok! TikTok is great at this. Once you watch a video all the way through, you will keep seeing posts by that same creator on your feed, even if you didn't bother to follow them. You'll also see similar content to what that creator has posted, what you liked, what you engaged with. The point is to keep you on the app. But the problem is that life is not lived in ninety-second clips. While we are going down the rabbit hole and consuming ever more content in the form of two- and three-minute videos, our time is still being taken from us, our energy is still being taken from us, and so is our understanding. Too many of us believe that we can receive everything that we need to know in a two- or three-minute clip and forget that a clip is often just a portion of a larger conversation. These clips lack context, and so we continually see things without the benefit of nuance.

CELEBS BE TALKING

I feel like Gabrielle Union and Dwayne Wade stay making the folk talk. But I wanna talk about a video that went viral in 2023. In the first half of 2023, Gabrielle Union did an interview where she talked about splitting things fifty-fifty with her hubby in addition to talking about monetary insecurities. That little forty-something-second clip went viral, and people started calling her all kinds of foolish things for participating in a fifty-fifty situation, saying that Dwayne Wade *obviously* is not a good husband if he would allow his wife to feel financially insecure in his presence. It was concluded that this was a display of a fuckboi attitude and a bad marriage. All that from *forty-something seconds*. Everybody drew a conclusion. But how many people actually watched the entire interview so that they could have context? See, here's the thing when we see things on social media, or even when we see things on TV: the things you see are often lacking in context. The kicker is the lack of context still impacts our understanding of ourselves.

Our self-concept is impacted because we are trying to find ourselves in the clip that we watched. How we find ourselves in the media and what we see in the comments can often inspire us to feel either great or bad, bolstered or shameful about ourselves. And if it's shame that we're feeling, then that shame prompts us to hide—not just from ourselves but from the people in our lives. It disrupts our connections with self and with others. While we are trying to hide those pieces that people already said that they hate, and trying to digest the dislikes of strangers, none of us properly minded our business—not the person talking shit on the internet and not the person trying to hide because of shame. I mean properly minding our business, minding what we need for ourselves and what we know about ourselves, because we failed to mind our business, we decided that their relationship is wrong not just for them, but for everybody. Because we've decided that it's wrong for them. We forget that you get to choose exactly how you show up in your relationship and that you and yours will have to pick the rules of your relationship.

Something similar happened with Tyler Perry around September 2023. He was on a podcast, and he mentioned something about light bills. And, of course, it was taken out of the context in which he said it. So instead of hearing the part where he said you have to find a partner who can meet you at your worth, we're having a conversation about partners who can meet us at our *net* worth. Those are not the same thing. Because if you recall earlier, I already told you that your worth as a human being is not determined by what's in your bank account. It is not determined by the job you have, the house you live in, or the car you drive. It is inherent to *you*. Finding someone whose energy matches your energy, I think, will often lead you to someone who financially is where you would like or need them to be as well, but damn if we didn't take that shit all around! It was clickbait. It was outrage bait. It diverted our eyes to maintain our attention, keeping us on the app by keeping us away from ourselves. We watch and listen to content, thinking that we will learn something about ourselves. But because we are getting content without context, we only hone our ability to react and not respond. We end up essentializing and generalizing concepts made for one person to everyone, and we sprinkle-sprinkle in a deluge of shit that doesn't even apply as a result. The sprinkling of information and the seeking of sprinkled information often means that we are not getting the full context. We take in opinions on social media, but forget to seek for ourselves as well as forget the context of our own lives. Conscious Lee (@theconsciouslee on Instagram and TikTok) is constantly telling us "research over me-search," but are you actually doing the research? Are we just trusting people on social media and forgetting where we are in life? Never forget that everybody has an agenda, including the folk you follow.

You Picking Up What I'm Putting Down?: Understanding the Goal of Social Media, Headlines, and Clickbait (Outrage Bait)

We know that the social media apps we use have an agenda, and we know that various media outlets also have a goal, but what we forget is that so do the people who are creating content. The goals that content creators have may very much be misaligned with your goal(s), which is why we have to practice curating the content we consume and consider our why.

So, how do you curate your social media (and general media) intake? You do the research. Consider what you know about yourself, where you are, what you need, and what you can handle—which will change over time. Because if you're in a space where you don't know yourself, having somebody else tell you who you should be is not going to be helpful. If you are in a space of low self-esteem, watching a bunch of videos dropped by a certain-looking individual or individuals is not going to help you.

✐ JOURNAL WORK

So, your homework for this section is to actually consider who you are following. I want you to pick an app—just one to start with—that you are going to curate. Next, I want you to go through and take stock of who you follow. How many people are you following? Who are you following? In what ways do they feed you? Because, make no mistake, you are consuming, which means you are being fed. And sometimes we are consumed by the very thing that we are consuming. So, I want you to be honest with yourself. What are you really looking at? What are you really taking in, and is that really what you need? Is it what you want? Is there a value match for you? Does it cross your boundaries so that you can stay in the know? Because let's be real, most of us have FOMO. I think that a lot of people will talk shit about things like The Shade Room (a celebrity news site) all day long and still follow it because we want to know what's going on.

They do say ignorance is bliss, but I don't think we know how to be happy. I think that we know how to be outraged, and I think we know how to be incensed. I think we know how to be bewildered. I think that we know how to create a life where we are constantly having our emotions strummed like a fucking guitar by a media outlet that simply wants your clicks, your eyes, and your money. These media outlets want you to pay attention to their stories, so they will say things in the wrong way. They will imply things that need never be implied. They will say things that are damn near untrue just to get you there. But the question is: Does it go against your agenda for your mental health? For your well-being? For your connection to self? So, start with one app, and when you're ready, expand that curating eye to other platforms.

Part two of this work is honestly noting how much time you're spending on social media. Now, most phones have settings that will tell you where you're spending your time, which apps you're on the most, and how much time you spent there each day in a week. I want you to do the same thing. Check how much time you spend there, because to me, time spent is like money spent. Where you spend most of your time and attention is where your energy flows. So, if you spend most of your time on social media, the energy is flowing there; you're getting, you're collecting, you're being consumed by, and you are consuming what is there. So, if it's there, consider what you're getting in return for your time and energy.

GET OFF OF MY PHONE!

One of the strategies that I personally have employed in order to get my life back from the clutches of TikTok and other apps—because, baby, they took me—was turning on the application features that allow them to track the time I'm spending there. To set my limit, I had to determine how much time I really *wanted* to be spending on these apps, which for me was no more than ten hours during the work week (weekends are fair game). So, you know, the personal tea is that all of my social media apps now have limits for the time I can spend on them. Instagram allows me an hour a day. TikTok allows me two hours a day. But I want you to consider this: Out of the twenty-four hours in your day, what percentage of that time belongs to social media? Are you comfortable when you know the math? When you know how much time you're spending? Does that match your values? Does it match what you know about yourself and what you want for yourself? I know what I wanted for myself was to read every book in my little library. I have close to three hundred physical books, most of them have been read. A lot of them have not been read. And I realized that I could probably read more books…if I spent less time on social media.

For me, it was about the trade-off. I've learned that, if I am overscheduled, I will get overwhelmed and become anxious, so I created a daily schedule for myself that automatically has space built in for things that bring me pleasure or give me rest—because, as Tricia Hershey from the Nap Ministry tells us, *rest is resistance*. My schedule also has a place for my goals, where my future self is considered in the here and now. This all started when I was trying to figure out how I never had time to read. How could I not have time to read, but I had time to be on social media for four or five hours a day? That was where the limitation of social media came from, realizing that I did not have a value that matched wanting to spend so much time on social media like that. But I did have a value that said I wanted to live my life, not watch other people live theirs, nor watch others record their imitations of life for the internet. I'm not saying social media and those videos are without worth and are not valuable, because it also gave me what I needed when I needed it, but I am saying that when it was time to let it go, it was time to let it go. It was time for me to get real, to get lit(erate) about me, to know more about me, and to know more about me as it related to media and how much I was consuming.

I also limited how much TV I was watching. Certain shows were activating me to the point of gratuitous anxiety. It took me a while to realize it. I said, "Self, you're a therapist. Do you need this shit in your life right now?" And since my answer was no, I stopped watching certain TV shows. I can appreciate what they offer, but them plots had me having palpitations despite the fact that I know they're fake. I just didn't need to consume it. I needed to consume something else. This was at a time in my life when my anxiety was at an all-time high, and I did *not* need more anxiety. I needed to find ways to soothe. I needed to practice what I needed for myself first. Only then was I able to reintegrate certain TV shows and movies into my life. But this is me being literate about me. Understanding how I was behaving and how the media was affecting my mental status and my health overall. I had to curate and limit so I could feel like I was on a healing path.

Healing Ain't Linear

Part of the problem with social media is that it shows us linear lives and healing. For example, it might show us that someone got a book or whatever, and then they did the work and were healed. While they might have been better overall, the idea that healing is linear is a lie, and one that harms us to the nth degree as we degrade ourselves for having setbacks.

THE SPACE TO GRIEVE

Your body undoubtedly has needs. And when things change, it is necessary for you to meet that need. This is why we have been discussing self-concept right alongside self-esteem. When you know yourself, when you can acknowledge your needs, you are not only better equipped to meet those needs, but you are also less likely to judge your needs against other people's needs.

Now, back to my client who said she was "dark, fat, and nappy." I remember one of the first things she said in our first session: "I just want to be better already." She was done with anxiety. She was done feeling depressed. And the thing is a lot of people come to therapy and say the same thing. Asking if we can just skip to the good part. The answer is no. You can't skip to the good part, because the healing we seek is in the journey. The healing is not the destination. It takes work to get there. Granted, when I was having anxiety attacks every two days, I also wanted to skip to the good part, but I knew that getting to the good part required me to do work in the here and now. Because, say it with me, *healing is not linear*. You are going to take incremental steps, maybe big baby steps, or bunny hops forward. Then you may end up taking one giant ass leap on an airplane backward. Healing may move in a general direction, but sometimes you're going to feel stalled. Sometimes you're going to feel like you went backward. Sometimes you're going to feel like you're never going to get wherever it is that you're thinking you want to go.

As you learn more about yourself, sometimes you find that there are things that you still need to address. This is why healing can't be linear. Because sometimes the thing that you need to address happened when you were eight. So, then you go back to your eight-year-old self and you love on them and you give what you can to that version of yourself and then you come back to you in the present time and continue on. You went backward so that you could go forward: *Sankofa*. You may then get to the next stage and realize some shit that went down when you were four years old is holding you back. So, you may go back to that version of you, then have to take a second check in with the eight-year-old you before you can adjust in the here and now.

☕ TEA TIME

I had a surgery in 2019, right before COVID hit, and it wasn't a linear process. Doctors will tell you that you'll be fine in two weeks, a whole lie. Either they lie or they don't understand healing or maybe they are using a "good enough" standard, who knows? But, usually, "good enough" simply means the point at which you're able to be a so-called "productive member of society" again, and being a productive member of society is just code for someone who is able to earn money and do labor. With the work I do as a therapist, it does not require me to move a lot. I sit my ass down. So according to the doctors, I would be healed in just two to three weeks. In reality, I had several days of crying, of being incapable of getting out of the bed, of being incapable of going up or down the stairs, of having to be in my bed, of feeling stuck in my room. It was a trauma-inducing time, because my body would not work the way that my mind was used to it working. So, my healing was further prolonged, because it took me a while to accept that my body had certain limitations at that moment. Even after my body was technically healed, the trauma lived on. Even now, I can feel the remnants of something off with my abdomen. Somebody else might feel a twinge in their elbow or knee when a storm is coming, got some ESP in their body parts. Meanwhile, is it completely healed if it's still getting that twinge? Or is this a new type of reality? Healing isn't linear. And I want us to know that and give ourselves the space to grieve.

Grieving is your body's way of knowing and expressing what it is feeling. And many of us have been taught that (1) you're supposed to get over things quickly, and (2) it's supposed to be a linear process. Many of us will talk about what we learned in Psych 101 way back in the day about Kübler-Ross and the stages of death and dying. What we forget about those stages is that they are nonlinear. Those stages can happen out of order. Just because you went through one stage doesn't mean you can't go back. It doesn't mean that you don't get stalled in one. I once had a client who got to anger in her healing process. And I was so excited for her, but she was not very excited. She was saying that she didn't want to be angry all the time. I simply told her that I love the anger. Anger tells me that now you understand—that your *body* understands—the level of injustice you've endured. Well, a month later when she was still angry, she was like, "This is not sustainable." I'm just like, "You have lived life with certain types of trauma and violations for over twenty years. Do you think that your anger should be done in one month?" She had to sit in that state that her body required. So, she was angry for a while; then she went back to being sad. And then she came back to anger. But she was angry probably for a good six months—probably for still trying to spare the feelings of those who had harmed her by maintaining her silence. It bothered her that she was so angry, but when she got to a place of accepting that anger for exactly what it was, and realized that the anger was nuanced, that she was angry at her family and she was angry with herself, that's when it left.

The Winter Whens of Taking Accountability

Taking accountability for ourselves means that we also risk having to accept liability when we fuck up—when we fuck up in other people's faces and especially when we fuck up in our own faces. It can be cold out there in these accountability streets. But when self-esteem is present—with an understanding of your needs, motivations, etc.—you are less likely to dip your beautiful form into the pool of shame that others want you to take a swim in. Shame is often said to be unproductive, and I agree. Shame-filled folk think *Something is wrong with me* or *I am broken*. This means we might try faking it and further disconnect from ourselves with avoidance and/or self-flagellation, or we could deny shameful instances even happen while we lash out and cause harm to the people who we don't want to see our secret shame.

Facing accountability with self-knowledge, literacy, and understanding of circumstances and messages within what we are consuming means, for many of us, that we have taken true responsibility. We understand that winter (our consequences) is coming. We stop seeing the world as "what you did to me" and also start seeing it for what we did to ourselves. We see the ways that we have compromised, allowed folk to overstay their welcome in our lives, and allowed the egregiously disrespectful to maintain access to us. In being literate, thoughtful, and "woke," you give responsibility to whom it belongs to, while placing blame where blame belongs. You take responsibility for your life, and that shit can feel hella fucking scary because I don't know about you, but I spend my life looking for the more adult adult. Yes, I'm an adult. But where's the adult adult? The adult that is more adult here than I am. I look for them. I will call my mom in a heartbeat off some stuff I already know. Because I need a more adult adult, an adult who has been adulting longer to tell me what she knows.

My momma and I, though we may look alike, didn't live the same life. I don't have any children. I got married much later. I did not skip countries. I didn't even really skip states. My mom's adult experiences are different than my own, and yet I still seek her or other adults out when I have a question. And sometimes I have to recognize that I'm only asking the question because I want someone else to take responsibility or share liability with me if something goes awry. Once I learned that, I realized that I was using it as an excuse not to move. Someone I thought was a friend told me that they didn't think my very first retreat was going to be a success. They told me everything that I was doing wrong. They told me what I should be doing if I actually wanted to achieve success. But my first retreat *was* a success. My goal always was to have one hundred percent attendance, but I also was just like, "You know what, let's go for a cool seventy percent." That's exactly what we got. We got seven people out of ten. We met the goal. My goal was to use this first retreat and play it like a game of spades, where the first hand bids itself. Where you use it as a learning opportunity because you know you got to play a couple more rounds so you got to get the three hundred. You don't give up just because you lose one hand. Because I didn't do it the way she did it. Because I was doing it in a way that I understood with what I knew I wanted to create and curate, for her, it looked wrong. To me, it looked right. Me seeking her out and me seeking her opinion was me trying to share liability. But, ultimately, I had to decide if I was going to allow her words to be the thing that stopped me. How often are you seeking someone to take responsibility for your life's choices? Even parents can only give us what they can. Some don't. Some won't. But ultimately, at some point you have to take what you have and keep it pushing.

When you take full account of yourself, when you mind your matter, when you place your mind over the matter of others, and know that yours is the only one you need to be looking at, you can change your life. We say, "Drink water. Mind our business," but we don't be doing that; we're not built that way. We want to mind everybody else's business, and social media certainly is not going to help us.

✍ JOURNAL WORK

I want you to take a moment and write a letter to yourself about the ways in which you haven't been taking responsibility for yourself. I want you to be honest. I also want you to write how you're going to take it back. I'll see you for our ending word.

Drink Water...

So, in this book, which is broken up into two parts, we talked about *mind over matter and minding our matter*. The first part informational, the second part instructional.

Per my last message: this book was not written for the sake of writing a book. The point of this book is to look at self-esteem intersectionally, specifically the intersections of self-esteem in your life. I am an operational definition girlie. What I mean by that is that when I understand a concept better, I can see how things fit together and how they may be taking my Black ass for a ride in life. My hope was that by breaking this book down into two parts, the knowing more and the doing more parts, that you can more clearly see the BS that has been between you and feeling yourself more fully. Why? Because you are the shit!

Personally, I think that loving ourselves and feeling ourselves is our default state. It's the garbage we get from families, the white supremacist delusion, the patriarchy, and more that gets in the way. That makes our glasses dirty. This book is to remind you how great you already are. To remind you that society doesn't get to dictate how you get to live in your body. Nothing says, "I love you," quite like destroying the system that took root within you.

My hope is that this shows you where the dirt is on your glasses, so you can choose how you deal with it. My hope is that your healing inspires others who get to be in your presence to divest from supremacy culture, as well as be inspired to start their healing journeys.

You made it to the end. You got here. You did it. You finished. Hopefully, there are some highlights. Hopefully, you got a good word or two. Hopefully, you learned something about yourself throughout the process. And hopefully, you took me seriously when I said not to do it by yourself.

This is a moment for you to look back. *Sankofa*, you know I'm into it. Where were you when you started reading this book, and where are you at this moment? Now, I understand that some of us may be on that speed-reading shit and will finish a book in about two minutes. And some of us take our time. Some of us read through once and then go back and do things on the second round—which was my recommendation. But the fact is you got to this point, and hopefully you came away with something.

⬙ JOURNAL WORK

Grab a journal and list ten ideas you have that you want to do something with. How did you deal with those things in the past? How have you been dealing with them in the here and now? How would you like to deal with them in your future? Because the future is cultivated by you—especially if you're taking responsibility for it and yourself. Especially if you're not allowing somebody else's narrative to dictate your life; especially if you're learning yourself so that *you* can love you, too.

My instructions for how to continue are simple:

1. **Step one:** Drink water.
2. **Step two:** Mind your business.

Take the time to learn more about yourself, to experiment, to try new things, to be able to definitively say what you like and don't like in various moments and know that you may like or dislike something in a later moment. Take time to understand the dynamics that have occurred in your family. Find the support that you need with the family that you create. With lovers and with friends.

Take the time to honestly look at your life and the values that you are living versus the values that you say you have, and consider how you can bridge the gap between what you're doing and what you would like to be doing. We don't change everything all at once, friend; no therapist would ever tell you to. It is an unsustainable practice. No therapist would tell you to just remove shit from your life without also having a replacement. Because holes and gaps get filled, and sometimes they get filled with bullshit. Even as we remove one bullshit thing, we add another, so consider one thing that you want to do in the next twenty-four hours. That you know you got, even if the thing you want to do is to get together a group of your girls and go through this book together and have a conversation about how you're going to support each other through work. Healing ain't linear. Grabbing rest is difficult or can be difficult; living a pleasure-filled life requires purpose and healing self-esteem, growing self-esteem. Being secure in one's self-esteem is work. The work is not always easy. The work is not always pleasant. But you have an opportunity to high-step into you. Into the version you are and love now, to the version of you that you yearn to be, be able to grieve past versions that got you to where you are and appreciate them, high-five them, hug them. Take lessons from them and apply those lessons to the you that you are in the moment and the one that you're going to be in a second. You are not alone in this journey.

Don't forget to visit the website and tell me tell me what you got. Send me a letter, an email, find and follow me on social media. I am @Dr.DonnaOriowo on Instagram and TikTok. If you remove the period, you will find me on X/Twitter. I can't promise to read every single one with my eyes. But I will keep them. I will refer to them. Hopefully I get to a mental/emotional space where I have created the time to one day open and respond to them.

All right, fine. Go do the work.

...AND MIND YOUR BUSINESS.

Acknowledgments

"If you want to go fast, go alone.
If you want to go far, go together."

Acknowledgments in books have always been weird to me. It feels just as performative as wishing a family member "Happy Burthdai" on social media when I could call them or pop up.

However, I recognize this for what it is, an out LOUD permanent acknowledgment of those who helped me get to this place. For the people who pushed me to go further and further, when I am a girl who likes the end to be here NOW.

In no particular order but with much love and gratitude in my heart, I want to thank all the people who got me here.

Thank you to my agent Ameerah at Serendipity Literary Agency—those random phone calls, pre-readings, and ramblings paid off into a finished book! Thank you, Kate, my editor, for getting lost in the pages when you were supposed to be critical and had to go back and read it again. LMAO. That will forever be a tickling moment!

Thank you to my sisters and my parents. Thank you to Mr.

BooThang.

I want to thank the people who taught me formally and informally. The people who love(d) me quietly and out loud. I want to thank all my pre-readers, the people who held my hand, the people who kicked my butt, and the folk who would tell all the people that something was coming before it was ever ready. LOL.

I want to thank Dr. Melissa Robinson-Brown, for reading the very first draft roughly written in a hotel room in Jamaica, those many years ago. I want to thank Rachel Okunubi for telling me about Dr. Joy, forward writer extraordinaire, who connected me with my agent Ameerah, who found my editor Kate Roddy at Sourcebooks, who pushed this manuscript further than I thought possible.

And I want to thank ME! I thank myself for cultivating patience, learning to ask for help, and not settling for being somewhere quickly when I could be surrounded by love and care.

And finally, I want to thank the Universe and God(dess) who are always listening and waiting for us to ask.

Notes

Chapter 1: What the Hell Is Self-Esteem, Anyway?

1   Karen Huffman, *Psychology in Action,* 7th ed. (Hoboken: Wiley, 2004), 466–467.

2   Barbara M. Newman and Philip R. Newman, *Development Through Life: A Psychosocial Approach,* 10th ed. (Cengage Learning, 2009), 258–260.

Chapter 2: What Makes up Self-Esteem?

1   Renata Marčič and Darja Grum, "Gender Differences in Self-Concept and Self-Esteem Components," *Studia Psychologica* 53, (2011): 373–384, https://www.studiapsychologica.com/uploads/MARCIC _SP_04_vol.53_2011_pp.373-384.pdf.

2   Glenn R. Schiraldi, *The Self-Esteem Workbook* (New Harbinger Publications, 2001), 19–35.

3   Schiraldi, *The Self-Esteem Workbook,* 19–35.

4   Enrique Burunat, "Love Is Not an Emotion," *Psychology* 7, (2016): 1883–1910, https://www.scirp.org/journal/paperinformation? paperid=72678.

5 Teju Ravilochn, "Could the Blackfoot Wisdom That Inspired Maslow Help Us Now?" Medium, April 4, 2021, https://gatherfor.medium.com/maslow-got-it-wrong-ae45d6217a8c.

Chapter 3: Do You VALUE Self-Esteem?

1 Michael P. Nichols, *Family Therapy: Concepts and Methods* (Pearson, 2010), 167–191.

2 Natalie Robehmed, "Men Have More Lines Than Women in Disney Movies, Rom-Coms and Every Other Genre," Forbes, April 8, 2016, https://www.forbes.com/sites/natalierobehmed/2016/04/08/men-have-more-lines-than-women-in-disney-movies-rom-coms-and-every-other-genre/?sh=6d22ba6321ee.

3 "The Wage Gap #IRL (In Real Life) for Women of Color: Groceries, Child Care and Student Loans," National Partnership for Women and Families, March 2024, https://nationalpartnership.org/wp-content/uploads/2023/02/quantifying-americas-gender-wage-gap.pdf.

4 Emma Hinchliffe and Nina Ajemian, "The Share of Women Running Global 500 Companies falls to just 5.6%," Fortune, August 5, 2024, https://fortune.com/2024/08/05/the-share-of-women-running-global-500-companies-falls-to-just-5-6/.

Chapter 4: What We Not Gon' Do!

1 "You're the Star of the Show with Main Character Syndrome," Cleveland Clinic, December 14, 2023, https://health.clevelandclinic.org/what-to-know-about-main-character-syndrome.

2 "Angela Davis and Nikki Giovanni's LIVE Discussion with GirlTrek,"

GirlTREK Movement, May 9, 2020, Youtube video, 1:48:02, https://
www.youtube.com/watch?v=esPHDvx_aZc.

3   Lexx James, "Ain't no teenage girl 'fast' enough to catch a grown
man who isn't attracted to children" Facebook, January 4, 2019,
https://www.facebook.com/Lexxthesexdoc/posts/pfbid02U
eJpQFdrfYAzomJGqoDvikBNTLXb6aztdBvWHhnAGB44DfFLo
Aqcbdz7xqRkEQ3hl?rdid=n5P5LKsqTddC6n6e.

4   Rachaell Davis, "New Study Shows Black Women Are Among the Most
EduatedGroupintheUnitedStates,"Essence,October27,2020,https://
www.essence.com/news/new-study-black-women-most-educated/.

5   "Issa Rae - 'I'm rooting for everybody black' - Full Emmy Red Carpet
interview," Variety, September 19, 2017, Youtube video, 3:02, https://
www.youtube.com/watch?v=WafoKj6MzcU.

Chapter 5: Sex and Self-Esteem

1   Evonne M. Hedgepeth and Joan Helmich, *Teaching about Sexuality
an HIV: Principles and Methods for Effective Education* (NYU
Press, 2000), 1–5.

2   Donna Oriowo, *Is It Easier For Her: Afro-Textured Hair and
Its Effects on Black Female Sexuality: A Mixed Methods
Approach,* (Widener University, 2016).

Chapter 6: Becoming the Bob the Builder of Boundaries

1   Henry Cloud and John Townsend, *Boundaries in Marriage:
Understanding the Choices That Make or Break Loving
Relationships,* (Zondervan, 1999), 18–19.

2   "Weaponized Incompetence," Psychology Today, Accessed January 11, 2024, https://www.psychologytoday.com/us/basics/weaponized-incompetence.

Chapter 7: Self-Talk Is Communication

1   Jon Michail, "Strong Nonverbal Skills Matter Now More Than Ever in This 'New Normal,'" Forbes, August 24, 2020, https://www.forbes.com/sites/forbescoachescouncil/2020/08/24/strong-nonverbal-skills-matter-now-more-than-ever-in-this-new-normal/?sh=5a6cd6415c61.

Chapter 8: Body Mapping Self-Esteem

1   Monique Deveaux, "Feminism and Empowerment: A Critical Reading of Foucault," Feminist Studies 20, no. 2 (1994), https://www.jstor.org/stable/3178151.

References and Resources

References

Adams, Elizabeth, et al., "Longitudinal Relations between Skin Tone and Self-Esteem in African American Girls." *Developmental Psychology* 56, no. 12 (2020): 2322–2330. https://doi.org/10.1037/dev0001123.

Advanced Psychology Services. "Help Your Child Develop These 10 Core Components of Self-Esteem." September 27, 2019. https://www.psy-ed.com/wpblog/components-of-self-esteem/.

Barowski, Janelle. "Self-Esteem Definition, Pillars, and Examples." Study.com. Updated November 21, 2023. https://study.com/learn/lesson/six-pillars-self-esteem-nathaniel-branden-theory-overview-examples.html.

Brown, Adrienne Maree. *Pleasure Activism: The Politics of Feeling Good.* AK Press, 2019.

Burunat, Enrique. "Love Is Not an Emotion." *Psychology* 7, (2016): 1883–1910. https://www.scirp.org/journal/paperinformation?paperid=72678.

Cleveland Clinic. "You're the Star of the Show with Main Character

Syndrome." December 14, 2023. https://health.clevelandclinic.org /what-to-know-about-main-character-syndrome.

Chapman, Gary. *The 5 Love Languages: The Secret to Love That Lasts*. Northfield Publishing, 1992.

Cherry, Kendra. "What Is Self-Esteem: Your Sense of Personal Worth or Value." Verywell Mind. December 5, 2023. https://www.verywell mind.com/what-is-self-esteem-2795868.

Cloud, Henry, and John Townsend. *Boundaries in Marriage: Understanding the Choices That Make or Break Loving Relationships*. Zondervan, 1999.

Cloud, Henry, and John Townsend. *Boundaries: When to Say Yes, How to Say No to Take Control of Your Life*. Zondervan, 2017.

Collins, Patricia Hill. *Black Feminist Thought: Knowledge, Consciousness, and the Politics of Empowerment*. Routledge, 2000.

Collins, Patricia Hill. *Black Sexual Politics: African Americans, Gender, and the New Racism*. Routledge, 2004.

Court, Andrew. "Attractive Women Brag about 'Pretty Privilege' and the Insane Benefits They Get." *New York Post*. January 5, 2022. https://nypost.com/2022/01/05/attractive-women-reveal-benefits -of-pretty-privilege/.

Deveaux, Monique. "Feminism and Empowerment: A Critical Reading of Foucault." *Feminist Studies* 20, no. 2 (1994). https://www.jstor .org/stable/3178151.

Fern, Jessica. *Polysecure: Attachment, Trauma, and Consensual Nonmonogamy*. Thornapple Press, 2020.

Feuerman, Marni. "Sternberg's Triangular Theory of Love." Verywell

Mind. March 27, 2023. https://www.verywellmind.com/types-of-love-we-experience-2303200.

Raypole, Crystal. "First Impressions Aren't Always Accurate: Countering the Horn Effect." Healthline, October 28, 2020. https://www.healthline.com/health/horn-effect.

Hershey, Tricia. *Rest Is Resistance: A Manifesto*. Hachette, 2022.

Huffman, Karen. *Psychology in Action*. 7th ed. Hoboken: Wiley, 2004, 466–467.

Johnson, Trilby. "3 Elements of Self-Esteem." *Thrive Global*. September 4, 2018. https://community.thriveglobal.com/info-trilby johnsontheconnective-com/.

Caskey, Johanna. "Fragile vs. Secure High Self-Esteem: Why the Ego Isn't Real Self-Esteem." LIFE Intelligence. February 17, 2021. https://www.lifeintelligence.io/blog/fragile-vs-secure-high-self-esteem-why-ego-isnt-real-self-esteem.

Marčič, Renata, and Darja Grum. "Gender Differences in Self-Concept and Self-Esteem Components." *Studia Psychologica* 53. (2011): 373–384. https://www.studiapsychologica.com/uploads/MARCIC_SP_04_vol.53_2011_pp.373-384.pdf.

Mayo Clinic. "Self-Esteem: Take Steps to Feel Better about Yourself." July 6, 2022. https://www.mayoclinic.org/healthy-lifestyle/adult-health/in-depth/self-esteem/art-20045374#.

McLeod, Saul. "Self-concept." CommonLit. 2008. https://www.commonlit.org/en/texts/self-concept.

Merriam-Webster. "Self-esteem." Accessed April 27, 2024. https://www.merriam-webster.com/dictionary/self-esteem.

Michail, Jon. "Strong Nonverbal Skills Matter Now More than Ever

in This 'New Normal.'" Forbes. August 24, 2020. https://www
.forbes.com/sites/forbescoachescouncil/2020/08/24/strong
-nonverbal-skills-matter-now-more-than-ever-in-this-new-normal
/?sh=5a6cd6415c61.

National Partnership for Women and Families. "The Wage Gap
#IRL (In Real Life) for Women of Color: Groceries, Child Care and
Student Loans." March 2024. https://nationalpartnership.org
/wp-content/uploads/2023/02/quantifying-americas-gender
-wage-gap.pdf.

Newman, Barbara M., and Philip R. Newman. *Development through
Life: A Psychosocial Approach*. 10th ed. Cengage Learning, 2009,
258–260.

Nichols, Michael P. *Family Therapy: Concepts and Methods*.
Pearson, 2010.

Oriowo, Donna. *Cocoa Butter & Hair Grease: A Self Love Journey
through Hair and Skin*. Self published, 2019.

Oriowo, Donna. *Is It Easier For Her: Afro-Textured Hair and
Its Effects on Black Female Sexuality: A Mixed Methods
Approach*. Widener University, 2016.

Oriowo, Donna. *#RelationshipGoals Guide*. Self-published, 2020.

Pena, Reyna Jacqueline. "Secure and Insecure High Self-Esteem and
Social Identity Affirmation in Response to Belongingness Threats."
Master's Thesis. Loyola University Chicago. 2013. https://ecommons.
luc.edu/cgi/viewcontent.cgi?article=2469&context=luc_theses.

Psychology Today. "Weaponized Incompetence." Accessed June 7,
2023. https://www.psychologytoday.com/us/basics/weaponized
-incompetence.

Ravilochn, Teju. "Could the Blackfoot Wisdom That Inspired Maslow Help Us Now?" Medium. April 4, 2021. https://gatherfor.medium .com/maslow-got-it-wrong-ae45d6217a8c.

Regan, Sarah. "The 8 Types of Love and How to Know Which One You're Feeling." MindBodyGreen. December 28, 2022. https://www.mind bodygreen.com/articles/types-of-love.

Robehmed, Natalie. "Men Have More Lines Than Women in Disney Movies, Rom-Coms and Every Other Genre." Forbes. April 8, 2016. https://www.forbes.com/sites/natalierobehmed/2016/04/08 /men-have-more-lines-than-women-in-disney-movies-rom-coms -and-every-other-genre/?sh=6d22ba6321ee.

Ruiz, Don Miguel. *The Four Agreements.* Amber-Allen Publishing, 2001.

Schenck, Laura. "Identify 7 Basic Self-Esteem Concepts." Mindfulness Muse. Accessed June 16, 2023. https://www.mindfulnessmuse.com /positive-psychology/identify-7-basic-self-esteem-concepts.

Schiraldi, Glenn R. *The Self-Esteem Workbook.* New Harbinger Publications, Inc., 2001.

Tawwab, Nedra Glover. *Set Boundaries, Find Peace: A Guide to Reclaiming Yourself.* Penguin Random House, 2021.

Taylor, Sonya. *The Body Is Not an Apology: The Power of Radical Self-Love.* Berrett-Koehler, 2018.

Warner, Judith, Nora Ellmann, and Diana Boesch. "The Women's Leadership Gap: Women's Leadership by the Numbers." Center for American Progress. November 20, 2018. https://www.american progress.org/article/womens-leadership-gap-2/.

Resources on the Benefits of Pleasure

Ferguson, Sian. "Does Masturbation Have Positive or Negative Effects on the Brain?" Healthline. January 24, 2024. https://www.health line.com/health/healthy-sex/masturbation-effects-on-brain.

Huizen, Jennifer. "How Does Masturbation Affect the Brain?" Medical News Today. February 9, 2023. https://www.medicalnewstoday .com/articles/masturbation-effects-on-brain.

Morris, Susan York. "Does Frequent Ejaculation Reduce Your Risk for Prostate Cancer?" Healthline. December 5, 2017. https://www.health line.com/health/prostate-cancer/ejaculation-prostate-cancer.

Oriowo, Donna. *30 Day Masturbation Guide*. Self-published, 2022.

Women's Health Network. "Health Benefits of Masturbation." Accessed March 20, 2022. https://www.womenshealthnetwork.com /sexual-health/health-benefits-of-masturbation/.

About the Author

Dr. Donna Oriowo (oreo-whoa!) LICSW, CST, is an award-winning DEI advocate, international speaker and certified sex and relationship therapist in the Washington D.C. metro area. Dr. Donna is the owner of private practice, AnnodRight, which specializes in working with Black women on issues related to colorism and texturism and its impacts on mental and sexual health. Dr. Donna specializes in working with Black women to feel Free, Fabulous, and F*cked! She is the author of *Cocoa Butter & Hair Grease: A Self Love Journey Through Hair and Skin* and the host of a weekly community space for Black women called *In My Black Feelings*. Dr. Donna collects inspiring quotes, eats donuts, loves pasta, travels to learn, gives COVID safe handshakes, warm hugs, and (figurative) knocks on the head.

Dr. Oriowo served as DEI Co-chair and Communications Steering Committee Chair for AASECT. She is a member of the Women of Color Sexual Health Network (WOCSHN). She can be found on social media @Dr.DonnaOriowo, or you can visit her on the interwebs at DonnaOriowo.com.